A Practical Guide to Child Observation

Christine Hobart and Jill Frankel

Stanley Thornes (Publishers) Ltd

First published in 1994 by:
Stanley Thornes (Publishers) Ltd
Ellenborough House
Wellington Street
CHELTENHAM
Glos. GL50 1YD
United Kingdom

A catalogue record for this book is available from the British Library.

ISBN 0 7487 1742 0

Typeset by Tech-Set, Gateshead, Tyne & Wear
Printed and bound by T J Press (Padstow) Ltd, Cornwall

About the Authors

The authors come from a background of Health Visiting and Nursery Teaching and worked together in Camden before meeting again at City and Islington College (previously North London College). They were part of a course team involved in the development of many innovative courses for the NNEB. Christine Hobart is now Programme Area Manager for Child and Social Care Courses. Jill Frankel has retired from full-time teaching, but is still actively interested in all areas of Child Development and Care.

Acknowledgements

The authors would like to thank colleagues and students in the Child and Social Care Programme Area at City and Islington College for their support and encouragement.

The authors and publishers are grateful to the following for granting permission to reproduce copyright material:

ERIC Clearinghouse on Elementary and Early Childhood Education (pages 35–36).

Hannah Mortimer (pages 84–86).

D.E. McClellan and L.G. Katz (page 87).

Sheffield LEA (1992), *Nursery Education: Guidelines for Curriculum, Organisation, Assessment, Sheffield.* Available from Early Childhood Education Centre, Stand House School, Queen Mary Road, Sheffield S2 1HX (pages 88–90).

Pam Lafferty, High/Scope UK, 190/192 Maple Road, London SE1 8HT (page 94).

High/Scope Educational Research Foundation, 600 North River Street, Ypsilanti, Michigan 48197, USA (pages 92–93, 95).

UK GROWTH STANDARDS, © Child Growth Foundation (percentile chart, page 98).

NNEB (page 111)

Maggie Murray/Format (cover photograph).

Contents

AN INTRODUCTION TO CHILD OBSERVATION

This chapter covers:
■ The professional role and responsibilities of the child-care practitioner
■ The student as scientist
■ Perception: the act of interpreting our senses
■ Objectivity and bias
■ Cultural bias
■ Feelings and anxieties

Students on various courses are asked to observe children in a meaningful way on a regular basis, building up a portfolio of observations and assessments which will lead to an understanding of the development and needs of children. Observing children, in this sense, is different to being alert and noticing what is happening around you. These observations have a focus and are carried out in order to plan for and assess children in a purposeful manner. This allows students to understand fully their own professional role as child-care practitioners, and gain a true insight into good practice in the workplace.

At college, you will be learning the theory of normal child development and growth and to understand children's needs. By the practice of closely observing children, you will integrate this theory with what you are observing in the placement. Further discussion in your group with other students, and your tutors, will allow you to see how they have observed similar situations. You will become aware of the great variety and range in the development and needs of children.

The professional role and responsibilities of the child-care practitioner

Throughout your course the concept of professional behaviour will be emphasised both in placement and in college. This touches every area of the work you do.

During the period of your course, as well as acquiring a body of knowledge, you will also reach an understanding of accepted professional behaviour and attitudes.

With regard to observations, you must be aware of your responsibility to recognise the rights of parents, colleagues and children. Observations play a part in helping you to gain knowledge and understanding, and you will learn to interpret your observations in such a way as to promote children's development and meet their needs.

You will share your observations with members of the child-care team, so as to enrich their knowledge of the children, whilst gaining insight from them into the children's development and behaviour. You may sometimes wish to share your observations with a child's parent/carer, who might be able to assist you with your assessment.

You will become aware of much confidential information concerning the children and their families. The amount of information disclosed to you will depend on what is necessary to meet the needs of the child, help you to function within the team and to gain a deeper understanding into working with families. All information that you receive, either written or verbal, is strictly confidential. You should never share it with your family and friends. Even your college tutors will not want you to reveal the identities of the children that you observe in your placement. Your observations should show awareness of and empathy with the needs of children and their families regardless of race, class, culture, religion, disability, gender, sexual orientation or age, both individually and in groups. You should show respect and interest in the customs, values and beliefs of all the children whom you observe.

The student as scientist

All scientists collect data to test hypotheses from which to construct or test theories. For example, a scientist wanting to find out why there are fewer butterflies in a certain area of England might well present a hypothesis that the reason is a change in the climate, as there is not as much vegetation around for the butterflies to feed on. She will then need to observe the habitat closely, regularly monitor the number of butterflies and compare the food supply with that of another area in which there are more butterflies. Having collected all these data, the scientist may be able to show that the data either support or disprove the hypothesis.

In the same way, using a scientific method, you will collect data on child development and behaviour which will allow you to either confirm preconceived ideas you might have had about children or to alter your

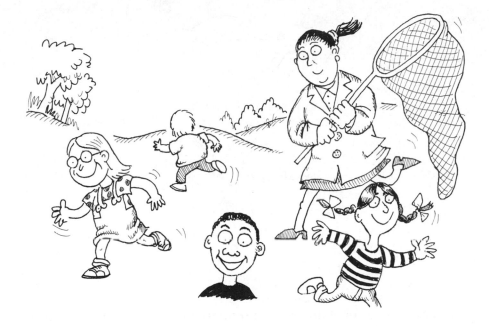

thinking in some areas. This approach demands objectivity – remaining detached from what you are observing and not allowing yourself to become involved as this may lead you to influence the outcome. This is not always easy as we are inclined to make emotional responses to children, but as time goes on you will learn to stand back and be objective in your observations.

Perception: the act of interpreting our senses

Perception is more than just seeing. It is our individual interpretation of what we see, hear, taste, smell and touch.

Look at the drawing on page 4. What do you see? Perhaps some of the students in your group will see a different person from the one you see. It is not always easy to rely on our eyes. How do we know that what we see exists? Do we introduce things from our imagination? For example, after a hold-up in a bank, the police will question the eye-witnesses as to what happened and what the robbers looked like. In general, no two descriptions are ever completely the same. People's perceptions are coloured by their past experiences, expectations, desire to please, possible fears and anxieties, and even last night's television viewing.

Trying to observe children objectively, so that you are able to convey your data clearly to other people in a way that they can understand,

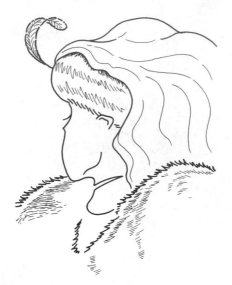

sometimes seems an almost insurmountable task. However, as in every other area of observation skills, you will progress in time and with practice. Often what is important to you can dominate the observation. You must take care not to generalise from your own individual experiences and expectations when observing children. Your interpretation of any observation needs to be based on the knowledge and understanding that you are gaining in your college work and in your work with children.

Activities

1 Sit down with two or three other people to watch a particular current affairs programme. Write down what you see as the six most important points made during the programme. Compare your lists. Did you all agree on the most important points? Did your lists vary? Why do you think this was?

2 If you are part of a class group, ask two students to role play a child-care practitioner reading to a child. The rest of the group will record what is happening. Read out your observations.
Did all the members of the group have similar recordings?

Objectivity and bias

Many factors might affect your observations. Preconceived ideas about the character or competence of individual children may influence your record keeping. Expecting a child to succeed in a task may prevent you recording accurately a lack of attainment. Knowing a child to come from an apparently happy and stable home might lead you to reject an observation showing a child at risk.

The familiarity of the setting aids objectivity. A child observed playing while waiting for a dental appointment would possibly not be as relaxed as a child playing in the familiar surroundings of the placement or the home.

Environmental factors, such as sudden hot and sticky weather or rain for days at a time, may well cause behaviour which is unusual, and should be noted in any observation. Difference in noise levels is unsettling for everyone, children and observer alike. Changes in routines, such as outings or visitors or staff changes, must also be recorded.

You must be sure that your observations are always a true record of what is taking place and that you are not tempted to add anything which might make them more interesting and easier to interpret. If you are assessing children's physical skills, such as the ability to skip, you must ensure that you ask them to do so in a neutral fashion and that you ask all the children in the same way.

If you are having difficulty in always being objective and being sure that you do not demonstrate any bias, discuss this with your supervisor. Some supervisors might find the opportunity to observe a child at the same time as you, comparing records afterwards. This may help you to look at children and situations with more objectivity in the future.

You may find yourself working in the same placement room as another student, and this might help you to check the reliability of your observations by both of you observing the same child at the same time and using the same technique. If 85 to 90% of your recording agrees, it can be seen to be reliable.

Cultural bias

You also need to be aware that many of the children you observe may have been brought up in a different culture from your own, which may have different expectations of children's behaviour. For example, a child who never says 'Thank you' when offered help might not have a word for this in his or her heritage language. Some children may dislike messy play as this has been positively discouraged at home; others may be very articulate as they have spent a great deal of time with adults. Yet again, some children from another culture will not look an adult in the eye as this is seen as disrespectful.

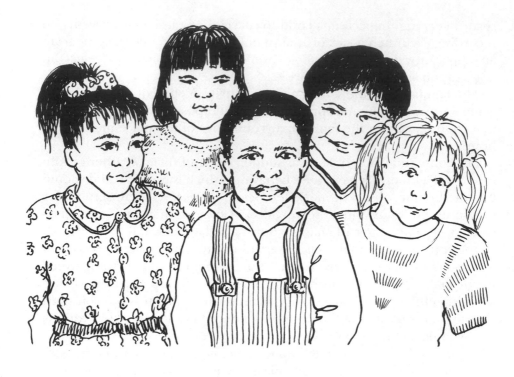

Activity
In groups of four, identify five different cultures and compare possible differences in family size, moral codes, diet, eating patterns and dress. Speculate how some of this knowledge might have an impact on your observations and interpretations.

The greater the understanding and knowledge that you have of other cultures the less likely you are to make value judgements based on your own upbringing and background. The practice of reading and discussing your observations in class will help you to become more aware. What we choose to observe is a matter of personal bias. Some people might be more interested in language development and record many examples of conversations with children, whilst others might concentrate on social development, recording friendships and social skills. To complete a satisfactory file, a whole range of observations need to be recorded, as you will see from the matrices on pages 110 and 111.

An observation is simply a sample of behaviour or development and you must be careful not to use it to plan for the child until you have confirmed your findings by doing several more observations. One observation will never give you a total picture.

Feelings and anxieties

It is quite natural to feel anxious and apprehensive at the start of a new course and, in particular, at the thought of being asked to do observations. Past students may have taken pleasure in telling you how complicated they are. With the help of your tutor and placement supervisor, you will soon make progress and even enjoy using various techniques. Observing children in the placement will help you understand the theory of child development and care, and is the best way of integrating theory with practical work.

You may have been brought up not to stare at people, and certainly not to write down things about them in their presence or to make comments about their behaviour. Some students will feel that observing children is intrusive and feel awkward recording what they see. However, you will be working within strict professional codes of behaviour and within the bounds of confidentiality. If you have these worries, talk frankly about them to your tutor. You will be reassured that these observations are often put to very good use, allowing supervisors to promote the development of the children in their care and to ensure that all their needs are met.

It is possible you may see an example of bad practice and wonder whether to record this or not. In all cases the observations should be about the child, or group, that you are watching, and bad practice only recorded if the child or children react to it. For example, you might record that a group of children were sitting at the dinner table for fifteen minutes before the meal arrived, having taken an equally long time to wash their hands and get ready. You might feel that a lot of time had been wasted, but it is the children's reaction to the situation that is important. Most supervisors, being professionals, will react well to constructive criticism, but if you have any real concerns you would obviously discuss the matter first with your college tutor.

You may find it very worrying if you record something about a child which might reflect on the parent/carer or the child's family; for example, a child who is very upset because he or she has not been collected from the nursery on time. Parent/carers have a right to see any observations about their children, and you must always keep this in mind. Your supervisor will give you guidance on this.

Very occasionally, through language samples or observation of behaviour, students identify children who may be being abused in some way. This concern must be shared immediately with your supervisor, who will take the appropriate action. You should also discuss this with your tutor.

2 *WHY WE OBSERVE CHILDREN*

This chapter covers:
■ **Integrating theory with practice**
■ **Normal child development and growth**
■ **Understanding children's needs**
■ **Social interaction with children and adults**
■ **Changes in behaviour**
■ **Health care and safety**
■ **Future planning**
■ **Identifying good practice**

Integrating theory with practice

'I hear: I forget. I see: I remember. I do: I understand'
(Chinese saying)

In college your tutors will be teaching theories of child development, education, health and childcare within a framework of social studies. Instead of learning this in a vacuum, you are fortunate in spending a great deal of time observing children and practising your skills along with your ever increasing knowledge. The exercise of observing and assessing children formalises the link between theory and practice, so that you are able to demonstrate what you have learned about children in all areas. For example, your understanding of a child's readiness to reach out and grasp an object at about 4 months, will be confirmed when observing a child of this age.

Normal child development and growth

Many of your observations will be about normal child development and you will need to understand very well how children develop in several areas.

- **Physical development:** this is divided into gross motor development – how children grow and acquire physical skills, from gaining head control to full agility – and fine motor development linked with vision and hand–eye co-ordination, such as threading beads.
- **Intellectual/cognitive development:** the development of children's ability to think and learn through interacting with their senses and experiences.
- **Language development:** from the first cry, through the growth of verbal communication skills, to true speech and understanding.
- **Emotional development:** from initial total dependence to full independence and autonomy.
- **Social development:** from close bonding to full and rich relationships with a complex network of children and adults.
- **Moral/spiritual and aesthetic development:** through socialisation, children develop a set of values and codes of behaviour and an awareness of beauty in the environment.

Many people have attempted to chart and record expected normal development, following observations of a large sample of children over long periods of time. It is important that you understand that there is a range and sequence of normal development and that not all children acquire skills according to 'the book'. For example, in possibly the most used book, Mary Sheridan's *Children's Developmental Progress from Birth to Five Years*, children are shown as walking alone at 15 months, whereas many of you will know children who walk much earlier than this. This could be because Sheridan's work was done mainly with white children in the 1950s, when many children were confined to cots and play pens for a longer period of time than children today, for whom there is greater emphasis on stimulation and play. Some children may show accelerated development in one area, whilst remaining on a plateau in another. For example, a child who is speaking in sentences at 18 months, may, at the same time, have difficulty in co-ordination.

One of the reasons for fully understanding normal development is to make you aware of development outside the norm and whether such development is advanced or delayed. This can only be detected through detailed objective observations.

In the appendix on page 114, we have devised a broad outline of normal development to help you with your observations. This is by no means the definitive text in this area and you will need to do a great deal of reading and be advised by your tutors so as to gain a full understanding.

Understanding children's needs

All animals have basic needs. Children, as human animals, are no exception.

Children's needs

Love	Children need to receive affection and to form close relationships. Without emotional security, children find it hard to make loving relationships in later life.
Food	Children need an appropriate healthy, balanced diet to ensure optimum growth and development.
Shelter	Children need to be sheltered from a hostile environment, to be adequately housed, to be suitably clothed and to be kept safe from injury and disease.
Stimulation	Children need the opportunity to play, to move around freely with safety so as to explore the environment and learn from their experiences.

Activity
The table above shows children's basic needs. What else do you think children might have a right to? What is the difference between needs and rights?

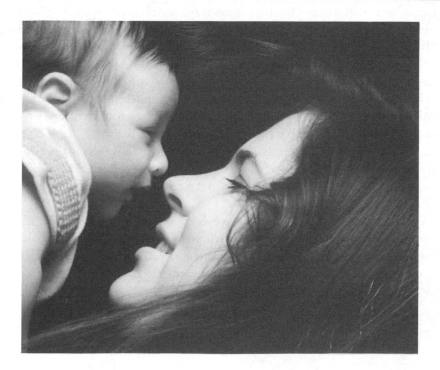

It is important that you understand the needs of children and become sensitive and perceptive in meeting these needs or in assisting parent/carers to do so. By recording objective observations you learn in a practical way how to become aware of these needs and how to meet them. For example, your observation of a child who drinks a great deal of milk in the placement, whilst often rejecting his or her dinner, might prompt your supervisor to discuss this with the child's parent/carers. At another time you might record a child who is reluctant to use the outside play area. This could lead to you finding out the cause of this and helping the child to overcome his or her fears.

Social interaction with children and adults

Promoting good social relationships is an important part of the child-care practitioner's role. It will start with supporting the bonding between baby and mother right through to sorting out peer group rivalry among 7-year-olds. It is only by closely recording the social interactions which are taking place that you gain an understanding of children's needs in this area and become able to help them establish good relationships. Children's rapport with the adults in the team will show you what is good practice, and help you to establish your own relationships with children.

Changes in behaviour

Systematic recording of observations will enable you to identify behaviour patterns and allow you to see behavioural changes in a child. Careful observations are useful in this case as the change in behaviour might have a physical cause, such as the onset of illness, or it might be an emotional response to family problems or changes.

You need to understand that all children are individuals and will behave and react differently in similar situations. Through detailed observation, you will be able to predict individual behaviour and reactions to situations, for example understanding that one child would be fearless on a new climbing frame, whilst another would hold back. You should respect both reactions.

Health care and safety

Making sure that children have the freedom to explore their environment with safety is part of your role as a child-care practitioner. Observations will make you aware of any potential hazards in the children's immediate environment and allow you to protect them from danger. This will link in with your growing awareness of developmental stages, for example stairs, which are a hazard to a crawling baby, present a challenge to a toddler. Your observations and knowledge of children's health care needs will alert you to signs of ill health. This could be obvious if a child suddenly vomited or had a skin rash. A child who appeared more lethargic than usual would come to your notice through your routine observations of a lively active child.

> **Activity**
> Look through the accident record book in your placement. In your opinion, were any of these accidents avoidable? Is there a particular area where accidents occur frequently?

Future planning

Observations are never an end in themselves, but should be used to promote and extend children's development, fulfil any needs which are not being met, support children in establishing meaningful relationships, acknowledge and understand changes in behaviour and ensure a safe, happy and healthy environment. Identifying any concerns should lead to assessment and possible action either individually or as a staff team, and may lead to discussion and planning with parent/carers.

All establishments are now expected to keep detailed records and assessments of the children in their care, and you should see many different examples of how this is achieved.

Identifying good practice

Through observations you learn to identify good practice and become aware of your own role in seeing how other child-care practitioners meet the needs of children from many different backgrounds. The placement will benefit from your observations in the planning and reviewing of their practice. You will not only observe individual children but, by looking at groups of children, you will see different patterns of behaviour and the interactions of the individuals within the groups.

LEARNING RESOURCE
CENTRE

3 *HOW TO OBSERVE CHILDREN*

This chapter covers:
- Beginning the process
- Guidance from college
- Supervision in the placement
- Involving parent/carers
- Starting out
- General guidance
- The front page
- Interpretation
- Personal learning
- References
- Bibliography

Beginning the process

The time has come for you to write your first observation. One way of preparing yourself for this is to carry out the following activity.

Activity

With a friend visit a playground, local park, or supermarket – in fact, any place where you are sure to see children – and, having gained permission from the parent/carer, separately record one child's activity and behaviour for five minutes. After completion, discuss the following points with your friend:

- How did you feel? Anxious, silly, unsure of what onlookers may have thought, detached and objective, any other feelings?
- Were you trying to write too much, recording language, physical movements and emotional responses?
- Did other adults interrupt and distract you?
- Did the child stay in the same place for the allotted time?
- Did you have to move?
- Was it obvious what gender the child was?
- Were you aware of the heritage language?
- Approximately how old was the child?
- Was the child aware of you?

- Did you ask the parent/carers' permission first?
- Did you have enough paper?
- Did your pen run out of ink?
- Could you write quickly enough?
- Did your account of the child's activity agree with that of your friend?
- Were you able to make sense of what you had recorded?

Having carried out the above activity, you will now be aware of the complexity of carrying out clear objective observations on children. Do not be despondent; the more observations you do, the easier it will become. Your file at the end of the course will demonstrate the progress you have made.

Guidance from college

At the start of the course, your tutor will help you to prepare for recording your first observations. Throughout the course, you will look at different techniques and methods of assessment and your observations will contribute to the overall learning of the group. In addition to this, your tutor may well use some tutorial time to give personal advice.

Your collection of observations will be regularly submitted and assessed. As with all the new subject areas to which you are being introduced, you will become more knowledgeable and skilled as the course progresses.

Supervision in the placement

The person who is responsible for you in the placement will be aware of the number and range of observations you are required to carry out. The supervisor has the following responsibilities.
1   Inducting you into the placement routines and making you aware of the timetabling of events, both daily and weekly. This will help you to plan the best time to do your observations.
2   Giving you opportunities to get to know the children, and giving you the time to answer any questions you might have about them. You will need the dates of birth of all the children to put on your observations.
3   Agreeing times during the week when you will not be expected to take part in the placement activities so that you can do your observations, making sure that all the staff in the room know what you are attempting, so that you are less likely to be interrupted.

4 Reading your observations and signing that they are a true account of what took place. Nursery and school staff frequently have many demands made on them. Despite this, most supervisors find the time to discuss and comment on your work and help you to interpret what you have seen. This should help you to develop skills and techniques and allow you to understand the progress you are making.

As a student you will need to find out the general policy and procedures used by the placement staff to observe and assess children in their care so that you can enrich and add to their own file of assessments. This is often a useful time to ask for their equal opportunities policies, which you will need to study and adhere to. The placement will have rules and guidelines regarding confidentiality, which you must fully understand before you start any observations.

Involving parent/carers

The placement will have informed all the children's parent/carers that you will be writing observations about the children, governed by the rules of confidentiality. As you become more skilled, and with the approval of your supervisor, it is good practice occasionally to share these observations with the parent/carers. They might be able to help you understand the child better, to point out why their child behaved in an atypical fashion, and to make you more conversant with the child's cultural and social background. It would be quite impossible to do some types of observations, such as a child study, without the help of the parent/carer. It is enlightening for the parent/carers to see how someone outside the family views the child and his or her needs and achievements. Specific permission must be sought before taking photographs or using other material, such as work with the child's name on it, that would identify the child, as this would break the rules of confidentiality.

Involving parents will help you to assess the validity of your observations and interpretation; for example, a child who does not have the confidence to read in class might well be reading fluently at home, whilst enjoying a cuddle with his or her mother.

Always remember that the parent/carer knows the child best. Establishing a good relationship with the family can only be in the best interests of the child. It is now universally considered good practice to involve parent/carers in all aspects of the child's development and educational achievements, and all reports and assessments have to be available on request. This undoubtedly has led to more objective record keeping.

Starting out

Make sure that this is a convenient time for the rest of the placement team for you to attempt your first observation. As an observer, you will need to blend into the background, so as not to spoil the results of your observation. Avoid making eye contact with the children and any adults who might be involved in your observation. Sit as still as you can and avoid making unnecessary noises, such as rustling paper. Try not to appear involved in what you are observing, but look as if you are purely concentrating on your note taking.

Very few observations need the presence of an adult, particularly the observer, to interact with the child. You are there to study children's behaviour, needs and development. Occasionally, interaction with an adult makes an interesting observation, but only if it demonstrates something particular about the child.

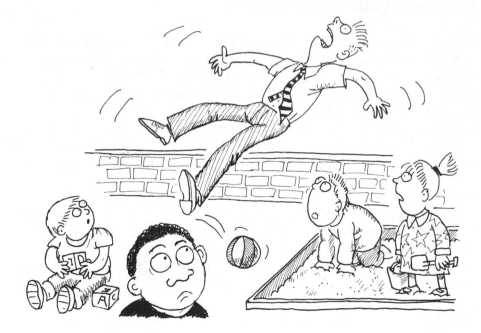

Decide to observe a particular child who, as far as you know, is well within the normal range of development and behaviour. Note down the date of birth, first name, and length of time the child has attended the placement. Taking a pen or pencil and a notebook, place yourself in an inconspicuous part of the area, where you have a good view of the child and/or activity you wish to observe, and where you can hear what the child is saying. Avoiding eye contact, concentrate solely on the child, rather than describing in detail the activity. If other children come up to you and ask what you are doing, just explain that you are doing something for college. If a child needs help with a task, direct him or her to someone else, if possible. If you find yourself becoming involved in an activity, stop your observation and try again later. If there is an emergency, when a child might be at risk, you must of course stop what you are doing and deal with it.

When you have completed your observations, you should spend two or three minutes reading them through to make sure they make sense and that you have all the information you need. You will then be able to write them up outside of placement time, feeling confident that you have completed a full record.

General guidance

Always keep a pencil or biro and a notebook in your pocket so that you are ready to record anything of interest that occurs. When you do your first observations, you will be well advised to look at one child, doing one activity, for a short time. As you become more skilled, you will use a variety of different techniques and be able to look at groups of children, which will help you to assess social interactions and relationships. Approximately a quarter of the observations in your completed file should be of groups.

Observations will also fall into various categories. Many observations that you do will be unplanned. An event will occur that you find interesting or that demonstrates an aspect of development that you wish to record; for example, a distressed child parting from a parent. Others will be planned by you; for example, your college might require you to set up an activity so that you can record a child's manipulative skills, for example with scissors. These observations will be of fairly short duration and you may or may not record that child again. You will also be asked to observe a child over a longer period of time, perhaps looking at several areas of development. These are called longitudinal or child studies. Occasionally, you may be required to record a quick impression of a child at a particular time, such as when he or she first joins a nursery group. This is sometimes called a snapshot observation and is also useful as a preliminary start to a series of observations on one child.

Many courses will ask for specific information, and this can be usefully done by having a common front page.

The front page

You will need to include the following information on a front page.

NUMBER AND DATE OF OBSERVATION

These are important for two reasons. Firstly, you may be asked to present your observation file to the moderators in date order, so that they can see a progression in your work. Secondly, you may forget to make a note of the age of the child/children you are observing. This will be easy to look up in the records if you record the date. The observation number is inserted in the box at the top left-hand corner of the page.

METHOD

Here you will note the technique you are using to record the observation, such as a written record, a checklist or a time sample, etc. These are explained in the next chapter.

AIM AND/OR REASON FOR OBSERVATION

If you have set up a particular activity, such as an interest table in order to observe cognitive and language development, this would be the *aim* of your observation, so you would put 'observing a 4-year-old using cognitive and language skills'.

Your tutor may have asked you to observe children's imaginative play by creating a hospital in the home corner. Then you might state as your aim 'observing imaginative play in 3-year-olds'.

If something occurs that you find interesting and you record it, you will need to give your *reason* for including it. For example, there may be an argument over sharing equipment and to your surprise the older child gives way and bursts into tears. You may go on to discover that the child is incubating chicken-pox, demonstrating how behaviour might change in an unwell child.

DETAILS OF SETTING

This refers to the actual place where the observation is recorded, for example the nursery class. Remember not to record the name of the establishment. On occasion, it might be illuminating to describe the wider context of the setting; for example, a rural nursery school might have a different philosophy to that of an inner urban nursery class.

IMMEDIATE CONTEXT

This would indicate exactly where the recording took place, for example the book corner. If you were recording language, it would usually be very different in the book corner to that used in the playground.

	Date:	Method:

Aim and/or reason for observation:

Details of setting:

Immediate context:

Time observation started:

Time observation finished:

Total number of adults in setting:

Total number of children in setting:

First name(s) of child(ren) being observed:

Age(s):

Gender(s):

Media used and justification (if necessary):

Supervisor's signature	Tutor's signature	Permission if applicable

Note that the box, top left, is used for recording the number or reference of your observation.

You may photocopy this sheet for your own use. © Stanley Thornes (Publishers) Ltd 1994.

TIMES

Noting the length of time of the observation is important for the reader's understanding of the event. The time of day might also be important. For example, a child crying for a parent/carer would have a different meaning early in the morning than at dinner time, as it is not unusual for some children to protest when separating from the parent/carer. On the other hand, it would cause more concern if it happened later in the day, possibly suggesting illness or a reaction to a problem at home or in the placement. If children are introduced to a new activity, it is usually found that they can understand it more easily when they are not tired, so the time of day might influence a child's response.

TOTAL NUMBER OF CHILDREN AND ADULTS IN SETTING

The reason you are asked to record this is to help you to evaluate your observation. For example, a child fiddling with his or her hair, isolated in the corner of the room, would show more worrying behaviour than if this were happening at story time in a large group and with an adult present. The impact of other children and adults on an observation obviously has a large influence.

FIRST NAMES OF CHILD/CHILDREN BEING OBSERVED

As a student, you should only use the first name of the child, or the initials. It would be a breach of confidentiality if you put the whole name. It is permissible to use a false name. For the same reason, you should never name placement staff or parent/carers, but put 'the teacher', 'the child-care practitioner' or the 'parent/carer'. Obviously, the name of the placement should never appear on your observations.

AGE(S)

Anyone reading your observation will want to know how old the subject is so that they can assess if the child is immature or advanced from the behaviour described. Years and months are usually written as follows: 2 years, 1 month – 2:1.

GENDER

Knowing if the child is male or female may be relevant to your evaluation. For example, identifying that wheeled equipment in the play area is dominated by the boys may lead the placement to discriminate positively to encourage the girls to have a turn first.

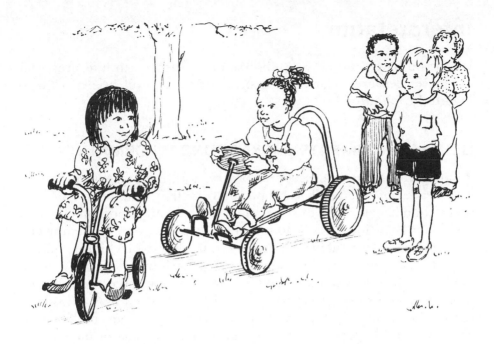

MEDIA USED AND JUSTIFICATION (IF NECESSARY)

Information may sometimes be presented in a more understandable way by the use of tapes, charts or other media, but you will need to justify their inclusion. Your tutors will give you guidance on this. For example, a photograph of a baby taking his or her first steps may illuminate your observation.

SIGNATURES

To verify that your observation is a true and accurate account, you will need to obtain the signatures of your supervisor and/or the parent/ carer, as well as that of your tutor in college.

In some circumstances, you may have needed to ask for specific permission, for example for recordings undertaken outside the placement. If in any doubt, discuss this with your supervisor or tutor.

The following page or pages will then contain the recording of your observation, whatever method or technique you have decided is appropriate. Finally, you will need to interpret your data. This is the part that most students find very difficult at first, but the value of doing an observation is to show what you have learnt from what you have observed, and to be able to use it to benefit the child.

Interpretation

When you have finished your observations you need to interpret what you have seen and heard. On many courses you will be expected to record the following.

GENERAL COMMENTS/BACKGROUND INFORMATION

Before you begin to interpret your observation, you may wish to inform your reader of relevant background information. The length of time that a child has attended the placement can have an important effect on his or her behaviour. If a child has only recently started at the nursery, note the date of arrival in your comment. It takes some children quite a while to settle into a new environment. The position of the child in the family may be relevant. Eldest children may be more used to adults, but more reluctant to leave the parent. Youngest children may be used to having their wishes anticipated for them by other members of the family and find it difficult to be independent. If the language of the child at home is different from that of the placement, the child might find life very confusing at first, and become frustrated and unable to express his or her needs. This could lead to aggression or crying.

It may be necessary to comment on the weather. Children who have been kept in all day because of driving rain may not behave in as cheerful a fashion as a group that has run around in the fresh air for some time. An unusual activity may have been set up by the placement. It might be necessary to describe this briefly to ensure understanding of your observation.

EVALUATION AND ASSESSMENT

A good way to start is to look at the aim of the observation and begin to link the evaluation with this. You must try not to make assumptions using words like 'I think' or 'perhaps'. Only comment on what you have actually seen. Reporting what your supervisors or other people might tell you about the child or the family background is not usually relevant to the observation, but if you are sure that it is you put 'Following discussion with the supervisor/parent/carer...' and then write what you have been told. Beware of making judgements based on race or gender stereotypes. The gender of the child may be relevant, but be careful not to express sexist attitudes: you should not be surprised if a girl enjoys rough play, or a boy wants to spend time quietly in the home corner. Not all black children will be tall for their age or advanced in locomotion skills.

Assess the child/children's skills, for example in the use of use of toys and equipment, language and behaviour, in relation to their age. Are those skills within the normal range, advanced, or immature? (You should consult various books on child development, information from your college, together with the charts shown in the appendix on the different ages and developmental norms; make comparisons with other children of the same age; discuss any difficulties with your placement supervisor.)

If the observation is of a child behaving in an unusual way, for example being very aggressive or anxious, upset or clinging, note whether this is typical of that child or very unusual. You or your supervisor may be able to suggest a possible reason for the behaviour.

Remember to be objective, never repeating hearsay, making unsupported value judgements, labelling children or being influenced by prior knowledge. Never personalise comments, for example making comparisons with your own children or other children well known to you.

You may find that you have not achieved your aim. This is acceptable if you explain why the aim has not been met.

POSSIBLE REFERRAL/COURSE OF ACTION

Owing to your observation, it may become clear to your supervisor that some action may need to be taken to satisfy the needs of the child you have observed. For example, the child may have a possible hearing loss and should be referred for medical assessment. You might discover that another child can read quite fluently and not even the parent/carer was fully aware of this. More appropriate encouragement and stimulus can then be provided. If you discover that girls in the nursery rarely use the large blocks, you can create a situation to encourage them in this area of play, which is valuable for their spatial and planning skills. You will be able to assess the value of the activity to the child.

Most of your observations will not necessitate a referral or a possible course of action.

Personal learning

You may well be able to demonstrate that theory learned in college has been observed in the practical setting. You might decide to follow this by doing another observation, perhaps using another technique. You may wish to repeat the activity to reinforce learning skills, varying part of the activity to promote a different outcome. You may also learn something about yourself and your attitudes. For example, you may consider a child to be very aggressive, and feel pleased if the child is absent on occasion. Once you have done a detailed observation, you might discover that the child is often provoked into fighting, being teased about living in an unorthodox household and wearing inadequate clothing. This may lead you to spend more time with the child, to consider ways of getting him or her to cope more appropriately with his or her feelings and to reassess your initial attitude.

References

Having completed your interpretation, it is necessary to indicate what has helped you to evaluate what you have observed. Whilst recording observations is a practical skill, it would not be possible for you to carry this out without some underpinning knowledge and understanding. This would include text books, magazine and newspaper articles, and college material. Any references given in your observation need to be cited in the body of the work.

Bibliography

Having completed your file you need to list all the references you have used.

4 OBSERVATION TECHNIQUES

The written record

When you first start observing children, you will most likely use the method referred to as a written record. This is the commonest type of observation technique, and may be used to record a naturally occurring event or a structured activity. You will probably use this technique several times before embarking on any other method. It is a description of an event unfolding in front of you, written in the present tense so that your reader can appreciate what is happening more easily.

ADVANTAGES

- You are using a skill which you practise every day and that is familiar to other people.
- Only a notebook and a pen or pencil are required.
- It can be carried out when convenient to all, with little preparation.

DISADVANTAGES

- Presentation may cause some observers anxiety.
- You may not be able to convey all you wish as the events are happening very quickly.
- The piece may be repetitious and boring, and could be conveyed better using a different technique.

| 15 | Date: 1.7.94 | Method: WRITTEN RECORD |

Aim and/or reason for observation:

To observe a four-year-old's drawing and to note the developmental stage.

Details of setting:

Nursery class.

Immediate context:

Table in art corner.

Time observation started: 10.05 am

Time observation finished: 10.17 am

Total number of adults in setting: 1

Total number of children in setting: 1

First name(s) of child(ren) being observed: Helen

Age(s): 4:2

Gender(s): F

Media used and justification (if necessary):

Supervisor's signature	Tutor's signature	Permission if applicable
A.N. Smith.	J. Jones	✓ E. Smythe

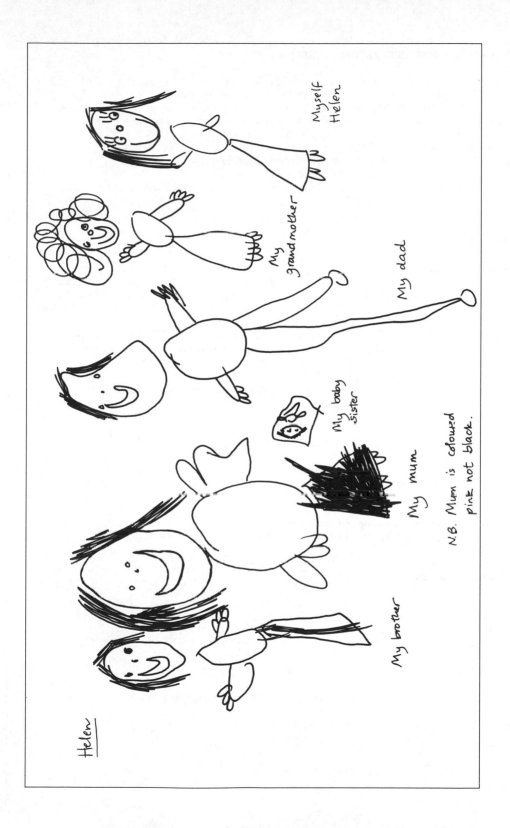

OBSERVATION (WRITTEN RECORD): HELEN

Helen is seated at one of the drawing tables with a pile of felt pens in front of her. She is bent over the table in concentration, her tongue sticking out of her mouth. She shows good co-ordination and manipulative skills with the pens, concentrating hard.
   Helen: 'My sister don't talk much.'
   Student: 'Babies don't say a lot, but they do cry.'
   Helen nods, and continues with her drawing.
   Helen: 'My Nan cuddles the baby all the time.'
   The drawing is now finished and Helen asks me to add the writing underneath each person.

INTERPRETATION

General comments
There has been a recent birth in Helen's family. Her drawing shows an extended family, including her grandmother, who lives with them.

Evaluation
Helen's drawing is mature for her age as she draws head, trunk, legs, arms and other features, including eyes, eyelashes and fingers. According to Sheridan (1991), this does not usually occur until at least 5 years of age. Although most of the details are included, Helen has not added the neck in any of her characters. According to Jacqueline Goodnow (1977), this usually develops last. However, Helen has passed the stage of joining the head directly on to the body, so showing an awareness of something connecting the head and the trunk. The drawings demonstrate an awareness of appropriate size.
   The drawing shows a child happy within her family environment, as all are smiling. Her remarks about her grandmother cuddling the baby shows that she may have some feeling of jealousy, but she is mature enough to express these in her speech.

Possible referral/course of action
Allow Helen more opportunities to talk about her feelings.

PERSONAL LEARNING

From doing this observation, I have learned how a 4-year-old can express her feelings in speech and in her drawings and the importance of the adults' response to this.

REFERENCES

Goodnow J., *Children's Drawings*, The Developing Child Series, Fontana, 1977.
Sheridan M., *Children's Developmental Progress from Birth to Five Years*, NFER, 1991.

Date: 22.7.94   Method: WRITTEN RECORD

Aim and/or reason for observation:

To observe a child who has recently learned to crawl.

Details of setting:

PRIVATE FAMILY HOME

Immediate context:

Sitting room

Time observation started: 3.00 p.m.

Time observation finished: 3.05 p.m.

Total number of adults in setting: 2

Total number of children in setting: 1

First name(s) of child(ren) being observed: ELEANOR

Age(s): 0:8

Gender(s): F

Media used and justification (if necessary):

Supervisor's signature	Tutor's signature	Permission if applicable
A.N. Smith.	J. Jones	M. Rigby (PARENT)

OBSERVATION (WRITTEN RECORD): ELEANOR

Eleanor is placed sitting on the carpet by her mother. Some of her toys are already on the carpet. Eleanor picks up a soft brick and squashes it between her fingers. She looks around the room and lets out a squeal and starts crawling.

Eleanor crawls underneath the table, a toy car is on the floor. She stretches her hand for it, but is unable to reach it. Eleanor looks up at her mother who says 'Go on, Eleanor, you can do it.'

Eleanor squeals again, and once again attempts to retrieve the car. This time she succeeds. She smiles as she places the car in her mouth.

INTERPRETATION

General comments
Eleanor is an only child who receives a great deal of attention, encouragement and stimulation from her parents.

Evaluation
Eleanor has recently learned to crawl and is thoroughly enjoying this stage of locomotive development. Once she got going, she moved steadily and quite speedily. She vocalised her intention of moving towards the car and responded to directions from her mother showing comprehension and determination.

She is at the sensori-motor stage of development, putting everything into her mouth. This is a normal way of exploring objects at her age, as noted by Catherine Lee (1984).

Possible referral/course of action
Suggest to her mother that she provide sufficient equipment to allow Eleanor to move on to the next stage of locomotive development, pulling to stand. Now that Eleanor is mobile, it is even more important to make sure that her immediate environment is safe and free from hazards, as emphasised by Dare and O'Donovan (1994).

PERSONAL LEARNING

I last saw Eleanor ten days ago and although she assumed the crawl position, she had not managed to move forward. I have learned how fast this stage of development can proceed. Her mobility made me aware of possible dangers in the home and how alert her mother will have to be.

REFERENCES

Dare A. and O'Donovan M., *A Practical Guide to Working with Babies*, Stanley Thornes (Publishers) Ltd, 1994.
Lee C., *The Growth and Development of Children*, Longman, 1984.

| 6 | Date: 22.3.94 | Method: WRITTEN RECORD |

Aim and/or reason for observation:

TO OBSERVE A GROUP OF CHILDREN INVOLVED IN LARGE CONSTRUCTION.

Details of setting:

INFANT CLASSROOM.

Immediate context:

CARPETED AREA.

Time observation started: 1.30 p.m.

Time observation finished: 1.45 p.m.

Total number of adults in setting: 1

Total number of children in setting: 5

First name(s) of child(ren) being observed:

	TANIA	PHILIP	SARAH	NATALIE	YOUNUS
Age(s):	7:1	6:4	7:1	7:0	6:9
Gender(s):	F	M	F	F	M

Media used and justification (if necessary):

Supervisor's signature	Tutor's signature	Permission if applicable
R. White.	J. Jones	✓

OBSERVATION (WRITTEN RECORD): TANIA, PHILIP, SARAH, NATALIE AND YOUNUS

Five children are sitting on small stools planning a construction.
   Philip: 'Here you are Tanya, you have this piece.' He hands her a long pole.
   Younus: 'Peep, peep.' He holds up a wheel.
   Tania to Sarah: 'That's not yours, O.K? You share with Natalie.'
   Natalie to Sarah: 'You share with me.'
   Tania picks up a piece of construction from the floor and passes it to Sarah.
   Tania: 'You use this, O.K?'
   Tania (looking at Philip): 'He's got more things.' She is referring to several pieces of construction surrounding Philip.
   Tania: 'I'm going to get over there now.' She moves over to Philip, taking her stool with her.
   Tania: 'I'm not your friend, Philip.'
   Philip. 'Why not, Tania?'
   Tania: 'Because you've got all the things by you, that's why.' Philip gets up from his stool and goes to sit on the carpet where Tania had been sitting.
   Harry, who is also doing a construction at the other end of the carpeted area, walks over to the group.
   Tania: 'Leave the pieces alone, we are going to use them.'
   Tania (loudly): 'Hey, look, watch, watch. Hey, look you guys.' The others look up at Tania. She passes a piece of cord through the holes in the model they were making.
   Tania: 'This could be the electric, because cars have electric.'
   Natalie: 'I can twist this around.'
   Tania looks and says: 'What's your name again? Mmmm Mmmm. Yes Natalie, you can do this.'

INTERPRETATION

General comments
All the children know each other well as they have progressed through Infant School together. They do not always work together, but they had been on a coach trip the day before and decided to build a model.
   Tania has three older brothers. She is the youngest by five years. Her mother says that she is very precious, being the only girl, and her brothers are very good with her.
   Younus enjoyed being part of the group. He has just returned from a long trip to India and has forgotten some of his English.

Evaluation
Tania literally dominated the whole activity, giving orders, demanding attention and at times seemed prepared to stop at nothing, including emotional blackmail, to get her own way. I was rather surprised that Philip gave in to her so readily, as I had supposed he was one of the leaders of the class group. According to Helen Bee (1989), most American research has shown that boys do dominate the play at this age, but she does warn of the dangers of stereotyping.
   The children interacted freely, concentrating well and carrying out their task, displaying manipulative and imaginative skills.

Possible referral/course of action
I shall watch and see if this group works together again. If Tania continues to dominate, it might be the time to intervene and help the others to be more assertive.

PERSONAL LEARNING

When I first made notes on this observation, I found myself describing Philip as having a 'domineering' personality. I now realise this was stereotyping and not an acceptable judgement. I also found myself speculating on why he allowed himself to be ordered around by Tania, who is a most attractive child, but decided that this had no part in an objective observation. This was reinforced by a handout at my college (1994) on stereotyping, objectivity and being non-judgemental.

REFERENCES

Bee H., *The Developing Child*, Harper & Row, 1989.
College Handout, 'How to make objective assessments', 1994.

Longitudinal studies

A longitudinal study takes place over a period of time. It can last a few weeks, or a year or more. The reason for doing these studies is to look at the progress of a child in one or more areas of development: for example, to study the locomotive skills of a baby from birth until 2 years, or to record a child's all-round development over a period of time, as in a child study. This will help you to have a more holistic approach, as you chart the developing skills of one particular child.

You need to have a clear idea of what you hope to achieve by carrying out this study and discuss this with your supervisor or college tutor. In general terms, you should choose a 'normal' child from a stable family which is unlikely to move away from the area and one to whom you can gain easy access. It is vital to discuss the project with the parents of the child, not only to gain their permission, but also, hopefully, their co-operation and participation. Many parents appreciate a copy of the finished study.

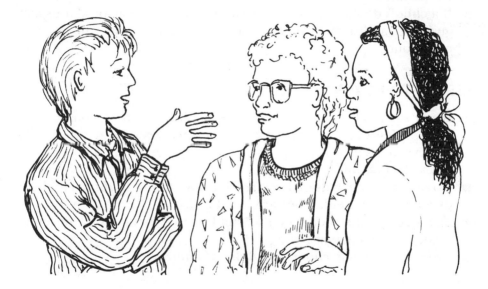

ADVANTAGES

- Getting to know the child and the background really well and being able to understand the influence of the family on the child's acquisition of skills.
- A better understanding of developmental norms and how some areas of development may be in advance of others at certain times.

- Closely recording developmental changes over a period of time.
- A detailed, more closely focused knowledge of one child, and an insight into the uniqueness of the individual.
- If through your observations you uncover an area of concern, you may be able to ensure that help is offered earlier than it might otherwise have been.
- The parents' participation allows them to have a better understanding of the child's needs.

DISADVANTAGES

- The baby or child might move away, or become ill. For these reasons, it is sensible to start initially with two children.
- The parents may find continuous observations rather irksome and relationships may become strained.
- Your objective observations may upset the parents.
- It may be easier to identify this child, thus raising issues of confidentiality.
- If a child's development or behaviour proves to be atypical, this may give you a distorted view of developmental norms and normal behaviour.

ISSUES TO BE AWARE OF

- Being so closely concerned with the family may cause conflict with your professional role. For example, you may exaggerate the child's achievements in order to please a family who have gone out of their way to be helpful.
- Do not record details that are irrelevant to the study of the child: for example, the parents' contraceptive history.
- You need to be aware of the child-rearing patterns of different cultures and religions.
- Avoid stereotyping children and their families.

ASSESSING PRESCHOOLERS DEVELOPMENT

Parents often ask how they can tell if their children's development is proceeding "normally". Preschool teachers and day care workers also ask for guidelines to help assess their pupils' progress. To address this problem, Dr Lilian G. Katz and her coauthors suggest that one way of getting a good picture of whether a child's development is going well is by looking carefully at his or her behaviour along the eleven dimensions outlined below. * One word of caution, however: the authors urge that any judgements about a child's progress should be made not on the basis of one or two days of observation, but rather on a longer period. A good general rule is that one week of observation for each year of the child's life will be sufficient for making an initial assessment. For example, if the child is three years old, observations should be conducted over a period of three weeks; four years old, for four weeks and so forth.

Sleeping

Does the child fall asleep and wake up rested, ready to get on with life? While occasional restlessness, nightmares, or grouchy mornings are normal, an average pattern of deep sleep resulting in morning eagerness is a good sign that the child finds life satisfying.

Eating

Does the child eat with appetite? Skipping meals or refusing food on occasion is normal; sometimes the child is too busy with other activities to welcome mealtime or perhaps is more thirsty than hungry at a given moment. However, a child who over a period of weeks eats compulsively or who constantly fusses about the menu is likely to have "got off on the wrong foot". The purpose of eating should be to fuel the system adequately in order to be able to get on with life; food should not dominate adult/child interaction. Keep in mind that children, like many adults, may eat a lot at one meal and hardly anything at the next. These fluctuations do not warrant comment or concern as long as there is reasonable balance in the nutrition obtained.

Toilet Habits

On the average, over a number of weeks, does the child have bowel and bladder control? The random "accident" is no cause for alarm, especially if there are obvious mitigating circumstances, such as excessive intake of liquids, intestinal upset, or simply absorption in ongoing activities to the point of disregarding such "irrelevancies". Persistent lack of control, on the other hand, may suggest the need for adult intervention.

Range of Affect

Does the child exhibit a range of emotions: joy, anger, sorrow, excitement, and so forth? A child whose emotions are of low intensity or whose affect is "flat" or unfluctuating – always angry always sour, always cheerful and enthusiastic – may be having difficulties. Within a range of emotions, the capacity for sadness, to use one example, indicates the ability to make use of correlate emotions: attachment and caring. Both are important signs of healthy development; the inability to experience them may signal the beginning of depression.

Variations in Play

Does the child's play vary over a period of weeks, with the addition of some new elements even though he or she may play with many of the same toys or materials? Increasing elaboration of the same play activities or engagement in a wide variety of activities indicates sufficient inner security to manipulate (literally, to "play with") the environment. If a child stereotypically engages in the same sequence of play, using the same elements in the same ways, he or she may be emotionally "stuck in neutral" and may be in need of temporary help.

Curiosity

Does the child occasionally exhibit curiosity and even mischief? A child who never pokes at the environment or never snoops into new territory – perhaps in fear of punishment or as a result of the over-development of conscience – may not be developing optimally. Curiosity signals a healthy search for boundaries.

* Written while Dr. Katz was Fulbright Visiting Professor, the paper "Assessing Preschoolers' Development" is coauthored by staff members of the Department of Child Development, Faculty of Home Science, M.S., University of Baroda, Gujarat, India. The full text of the paper from which this short report has been derived is available in ERIC as ED 226 857.

ERIC/EECE, College of Education, University of Illinois, 805 W. Pennsylvania Ave., Urbana. IL 61801

Acceptance of Authority

Does the child usually accept adult authority? Although the inability to yield to adults may constitute a problem, occasional resistance, assertion of personal desires, or expression of objections indicates healthy socialization. Always accepting adult demands and restrictions without a word may suggest excessive anxiety, fear, or perhaps a weakening of self-confidence.

Friendship

Can the child initiate, maintain, and enjoy a relationship with one or more other children? Playing alone some of the time is fine as long as the child is not doing so because of insufficient competence in relating to others. However, chronic reticence in making friends may create difficulties in the development of social competence or relationship building later on, and is cause for concern.

Interest

Is the child capable of sustained involvement and interest in something outside of himself or herself? Does the child's capacity for interest seem to be increasing to allow longer periods of involvement in activity, games, or play? The emphasis here is on "activities" rather than "passivities", such as television watching. A tendency toward increasing involvement in activities requiring a passive role or the persistent inability to see a project to completion may signal difficulties requiring adult intervention.

Spontaneous Affection

Does the child express spontaneous affection for one or more of those with whom he or she spends time? While demonstrations of affection vary among families and cultures, a child whose development is going well is likely on occasion to let others know that they are loved and to express the feeling that the world is a gratifying place. Excessive expressions of this kind, however, may signal doubts about the strength of attachment between adult and child, and may call for consideration.

Enjoyment of the "Good Things of Life"

Is the child capable of enjoying the potentially "good things of life", such as playing with others, going on picnics, exploring new places, and so forth? A child may have a specific problem – fear of insects or food dislikes, for example – but if the problem does not prevent the child from participating in and enjoying life, then it is reasonable to assume it will be outgrown.

The first three dimensions of development – sleeping, eating, and toilet habits – are particularly sensitive indicators of the child's development, since these the child alone controls. The remaining dimensions, more culture-bound and situationally determined, are still of great value in evaluation, since they are likely to represent important goals held for the child by both parents and teachers.

While the dimensions outlined above provide a useful place to begin in evaluation preschoolers' development, it is important to note that difficulties in any one of these categories, or even in several, are not automatic cause for alarm. Such problems should not be interpreted as signalling an irreversible trend; indeed, temporary difficulties often help those close to the child to understand when the child's situation does not match his or her emerging needs, thus assisting in the process of helping the child "get back on the right foot".

RELATED ERIC DOCUMENTS

Bagbahn, Marcia. *Language Development and Early Encounters with Written Language.* (ED 211 975, 24p).

Blevins, Belinda, and Cooper, Robert G., Jr. *The Development of the Ability to Make Transitive Inferences.* (ED 218 919, 11p.) 1981.

Burke, Julie, and Clark, Ruth Anne. *Construct System Development, Understanding of Strategic Choices, and the Quality of Persuasive Messages in Childhood and Adolescence.* (ED 210 727, 19p) 1981.

Katz, Phyllis A. *Development of Children's Racial Awareness and Intergroup Attitudes.* (ED 207 675, 55p) 1981.

Proctor, Adele. *Linguistic Input: A Comprehensive Bibliography.* (ED 222 282, 37P) 1982.

Wagner, Betty S. *Developmental Assessment of Infants and Toddlers in Child Care Programs.* (ED 223 565, 21p) 1982.

40 Date: 10.1.94   Method: Child Study
     to 4.2.94   Pre-schooler's assessment

Aim and/or reason for observation:

To observe and assess a 4-year-old child at nursery and through consultation with parents at home.

Details of setting:

Nursery class

Immediate context:

N/A

Time observation started:

Time observation finished: } Over 4 weeks

Total number of adults in setting: 2 in N.C.

Total number of children in setting: 20 in N.C.

First name(s) of child(ren) being observed: Martha

Age(s): 4.3

Gender(s): F

Media used and justification (if necessary):

Supervisor's signature	Tutor's signature	Permission if applicable
T. Weaver	M. Platt	✓

Pre-school assessment

Section: One

Sleeping

Week 1 Nursery	Home
Martha is usually full of energy in the nursery, needing no sleep during the day. It is rare to see Martha in a bad or upset mood; this week was typical of that. She has been happy most of the time, only showing signs of tiredness towards the end of the days.	At home Martha has no fixed bed time; it is variable depending on how tired she is. Sometimes she is very tired and can fall asleep as soon as she comes home from nursery, sometimes she is still awake at 22:00 hrs. Food has the effect of waking her up. Her mother tells me that at times it is a fight to keep her awake to eat but, as soon she has eaten, she is wide awake again. A late night does not always mean that she is tired the next day/evening.
Week 2	
As above. Only difference is that Martha now comes to the school at 08:00 hrs every day as her mother works in the Early Years Centre in the school.	On Sunday Martha was tired during the day and wanted to sleep. Martha's mother took her to the park and stopped her from sleeping. Martha perked up while in the park. In the evening she was still wide awake at 22:00 hrs; she couldn't sleep.
Week 3	
Martha was unusually tired on the Monday of this week, but was as usual the rest of the week.	Had a couple of late nights this week; other than that no change.
Week 4	
No change.	Nothing unusual.

Pre-school assessment

Section: Two

Eating

Week 1 Nursery	Home
Martha has eaten well this week at the nursery. There has been no refusal of any food and the amounts are of standard size. Martha never rushes to the dinner table and is finished eating at about the same time as the other children.	Martha has eaten well at home this week. This is standard for her. She has never been really fussy about anything and her appetite is normally good.
Week 2	
As above.	No change.
Week 3	
No change.	Martha's mother told me that Martha has food fads at times, going on to and off of some things. This week she was a little bit fussy about peanut butter. She no longer likes it.
Week 4	
No change.	No change.

Pre-school assessment

Section: Three

Toileting

Week 1 Nursery	Home
There have been no accidents at all in the nursery this week. Martha always goes to the toilet in good time while in the nursery.	Martha's mother tells me that Martha still has the occasional accident at home and that she wets the bed frequently.
Week 2	
As above.	No accidents this week, but has wet the bed on a couple of occasions.
Week 3	
No change.	No change.
Week 4	
No change.	No change.

Pre-school assessment

Section: Four

Range of effect

Week 1 Nursery	Home
Martha is usually a happy child in play and is always ready to socialise with adults. Martha shows concern and sadness if a playfriend is hurt or is crying. This week Martha accidentally ran over a child's ankle with a pram; she said sorry right away and displayed remorse for having hurt the other child.	Martha saw a child psychologist at one stage in her past. This was for uncontrollable rage or severe temper tantrums. By all accounts, these tantrums were brought on from moving house, or so the mother was led to believe by the psychologist. Other than this, at home Martha loves to mother younger children and babies and is normally happy.
Week 2	
Martha threw a tantrum this week in the nursery playground. This was because her mother and I were covering the sand pit and she wanted to help but was unable to. She was screaming and shouting at us. Her mother said that this was only because she (mum) was there and had it been myself and another person, this would not have taken place. This was the only occurrence.	Martha threw a tantrum at home when she wanted mum to join in with her game; mum was otherwise occupied.
Week 3	
Nothing to report.	No change.
Week 4	
Nothing to report.	Martha is more demanding of her mother's time since she has started working in the Early Years Centre, but has still a full range of affections.

Pre-school assessment

Section: Five

Variations in play

Week 1 Nursery	Home
Martha just loves toys of any description. She also enjoys playing without toys, for example climbing, running. This week has seen Martha riding a tricycle, pushing a pram, playing on a see-saw and working on the activity tables, both alone and with others.	Loves her toys and is possessive of them. She plays with all of them, not at the same time of course, but she never neglects any of them. Martha talks while playing alone, normally playing the part of the adult, telling the children to do various things. She likes her puzzles and books at home. She also paints and draws.
Week 2	
This week we introduced the use of woodwork tools and wood. Martha was keen to join in, and did. She also got involved with other children who were playing with a tent outside in the garden. This was used as 'a house' in their game. Martha used her imagination by 'going shopping' from the house.	No change at home.
Week 3	
Martha spent a lot of time in the Early Years Centre this week. She likes to play with the younger children.	Spends time playing with all her toys at home. This week is no exception.
Week 4	
No change.	No change.

Section: Six

Curiosity

Week 1 Nursery	Home
Martha wants to know about anything and everything. If a child is hurt, Martha is there to ask why and who. Martha is usually one of first to investigate anything new in the nursery. Nothing outstanding has happened this week.	Martha asks lots of why type questions at home; she is very inquisitive. She asks a lot of questions about her Gran, who died a little while ago. Martha thinks that her Gran now *lives* underground and that she still has a house there, still goes shopping, etc.
Week 2	
Martha was one of the first to investigate the woodwork table and asked what was being made, what the tools were called and what the vice was for, etc.	No change, nothing outstanding.
Week 3	
No change.	Still as curious as ever.
Week 4	
No change.	No change.

Pre-school assessment

Section: Seven

Acceptance of authority

Week 1 Nursery	Home
Usually Martha never argues with the adults in the nursery. She will ask why she has to do things, but always does them.	At home, it really depends on what is being asked of her. She 'will try it on' but knows how much she can get away with and when not to argue.
Week 2	
No change in attitude.	Nothing has changed at home.
Week 3	
No change.	No change.
Week 4	
No change.	No change.

Pre-school assessment

Section: Eight

Friendship

Week 1 Nursery	Home
Martha is usually an outgoing, friendly child who gets on with all the children in the nursery. Martha enjoys the company of others, but on occasion plays alone. Now and then Martha plays with the younger children and takes care of them.	Martha is not allowed out at present as the family live in a maisonette and it would be hard to supervise her. She still sees other children and makes friends easily, but not as much as before. She likes to play with children that are younger than herself and tends to try to mother them.
Week 2	
Martha has been playing with the children in the Early Years Room more than with her own peer group this week. She spends a lot of time there with her mother, but is not dependent on her.	No change.
Week 3	
Martha has spent equal time in both sections this week, but is still inclined to play with the younger children.	No change.
Week 4	
Same as above; no change.	No change.

Pre-school assessment

Section: Nine

Interest

Week 1 Nursery	Home
Martha is capable of involving herself in a particular task and seeing it through to the end. This is true of most things, unless it involves something that she dislikes. In these cases Martha tends to do a vanishing act. If Martha has any trouble with a task she asks for help, never giving up and walking away owing to lack of ability.	Attention span is variable at home. Likes to help with chores indoors, helping mum.
Week 2	
No change.	No change.
Week 3	
No change.	No change.
Week 4	
No change.	No change.

Pre-school assessment

Section: Ten

Spontaneous affection

Week 1 Nursery	Home
There has been no indication of spontaneous affection towards the adults in the nursery, but Martha does cuddle the younger children.	Martha always comes up and gives her parents hugs and cuddles out of the blue. Younger children and babies very rarely escape Martha's attention for very long. All babies that visit her family get cuddles and a kiss.
Week 2	
No change.	No change.
Week 3	
No change.	No change.
Week 4	
Nothing to report.	No change.

Pre-school assessment

Section: Eleven

'Good things in life'

Week 1 Nursery	Home
Martha never misses a chance to play with her friends, and seems to enjoy all special occasions. On Friday we went to the park, as we do most Fridays. Martha likes this.	Enjoys days out, playing with others. Martha does not go out much, but likes anything that is different. Hates spiders and flying insects, especially wasps and bees. However, this will not stop her enjoyment.
Week 2	
No change.	Nothing to report.
Week 3	
No change.	No change.
Week 4	
No change.	No change.

OBSERVATION (CHILD STUDY): MARTHA

INTERPRETATION

General Comments
Martha is an only child of average height and weight. She has red hair and green eyes. She speaks with a slight Irish accent. Martha's mother was very co-operative and gave me all the information about Martha's behaviour at home. I am most grateful.

Evaluation
I identified no areas of concern. Martha is a happy-go-lucky child who fits in well in the nursery group. Her sleeping pattern is irregular. However, she rarely seems affected by lack of sleep. She eats well and is willing to try new foods. Her bed wetting which, according to Pat Geraghty (1988) can occur in this age group, does not appear to upset her or her mother, and she never had an accident in the nursery during the day.

Emotionally Martha appears to be well-adjusted, displaying a full range of emotions. The occasional temper tantrum is expected at her age. Any behaviour problems which her mother reported her having at one stage seem to have disappeared. She rarely displays spontaneous affection towards adults other than her immediate family, but she kisses and cuddles all babies and younger children.

She enjoys all the play activities at the nursery and at home and joins in with great enjoyment. She responds well to new challenges. She enjoys all outings and special occasions. She perseveres well at the nursery, asking for help if she cannot manage on her own. She is inquisitive and asks appropriate questions. She accepts authority well, although may question orders at home. She gets on well with her peers, showing love and concern for younger children. She can play alone as well as with her peers.

In general, Martha is a happy, average 4-year-old showing the stage of development outlined by Mary Sheridan (1991) and College Handouts.

Possible referral/course of action
Not applicable.

PERSONAL LEARNING

I learned a great deal from this observation, especially from having such close links with Martha's parents. This gave me a very good insight into this child's behaviour and has given me a better understanding of 4-year-olds in general.

REFERENCES

Geraghty P., *Caring for Children*, Baillière Tindell, 1988
Sheridan M., *Children's Developmental Progress from Birth to Five Years*, NFER, 1991.
College Handouts on the 4-year-old.

Longitudinal Baby Observations

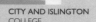

Your baby observations are a valuable and vitally important part of your NNEB Course. As a qualified Nursery Nurse you will be expected to have a sound knowledge of the health and development of babies, backed up by practical experience, as well as being conversant with all aspects of baby-care.

During the two years' training your work experience with young babies will be limited. It is, therefore, essential that you make full use of the opportunities afforded you by closely observing one particular baby. Your observations should reflect the baby's progress in the following areas:

1 **Motor Development**
   head control, rolling over, sitting, crawling, standing, furniture walking, walking

2 **Hand-Eye Co-ordination/Manipulative Skills**
   development of vision, grasping rattle, hand regard, reaching for objects, grasping cube, transfer of objects, immature and mature pincer grip

3 **Hearing and Language Development**
   response to sounds of differing pitch and loudness, turning to sound, locating sounds, development of sounds, e.g. 'a', 'm', 'b' through to first meaningful words, babbling, gurgling

4 **Social Development**
   smiling, recognising familiar people, e.g. parents and siblings, shyness with strangers, bathtime, feeding, weaning, finger feeding, drinking from cup

Baby observations should be carried out *at least* every two weeks and always by prior arrangement with the parent/carer. Your observations should always begin with *the baby's first name, age, date and title of the observation*. You will find the book by Neaum et al, *Babies and Young Children: Book 1 – Development 0-7* a helpful guide for your observations.

In addition to the developmental observations there are Health Screening Checks/Assessments which you are advised to make every effort to attend. It is the responsibility of each student to make the necessary arrangements with the baby's parent/carer for attendance at these check-ups. These examinations and assessments will include:

1 A medical examination and assessment at 6 weeks. Watch particularly for the testing of the primitive reflexes and the examination for congenital dislocation of the hip (CDH).

2 Hearing distraction test at 7 to 8 months. Permission from the Health Visitor will be needed to observe this test.

3 Possible developmental assessment at 9 months and/or 12 months according to the policy of the General Practitioner or Child Health Clinic.

It is also advisable that you attend at least one immunisation session. Details of illnesses or operations should be included in your observations. Permission from your Course Tutor must be sought for attendance at any examinations or assessments or immunisation session held during College time.

(M. O'Donovan)

Target child

The target child observation technique was invented as a tool to study concentration in pre-school children. This observation was developed in the 1970s as part of the Oxford Pre-school Research Project carried out by Kathy Sylva et al., and described in their book *Childwatching at Playgroup and Nursery School* (Grant Mcintyre, 1980). The purpose of the research was to find out which activities and settings furthered children's concentration, and which were merely 'passing time'.

You need to watch one particular child and see exactly what activity that child does over a set period of time, for about an hour. Any language use or social interaction is also noted. These two variables may or may not aid the child in concentrating on a particular task for a longer period.

This technique is a good example of a pre-coded way of collecting data. The group decided to use certain letters and symbols to denote:

- The child's task, be it art, or story-listening, or watching others with whom he or she was doing the task (known as the activity record)
- What he or she was saying and what was said to him or her (known as the language record)
- What materials he or she used
- What 'programme' was in force at the time of observation, for example was it free play or group story?
- Whether there were signs of commitment or challenge, such as pursed lips or intent gaze (ibid).

The Oxford group listed thirty different activity codes, such as gross motor play, art, and small-scale construction. These codes were devised specifically for the research and would be too complex and time consuming for general use in the placement. Nevertheless, you might find it an interesting way of closely observing one child, for example a child who used little language, or who did not appear to relate well to children or to adults. Any abbreviations you might use must be noted on your observation.

ADVANTAGES

- Gives a more focused example of a child's behaviour
- Allows observer to focus clearly on one child
- Freedom to add anything that seemed important to the child
- Shows areas most used by the child in the classroom
- Shows which setting promotes conversation.

DISADVANTAGES

- Codes have to be learned and need to be practised before use
- Need to develop ability to summarise precisely.

| 30 | Date: 16.6.94 | Method: TARGET CHILD PRECODED OBSERVATION |

Aim and/or reason for observation:

To detect any possible change in behaviour due to birth of new baby.

Details of setting:

Nursery class.

Immediate context:

N/A

Time observation started: 10.35 a.m.

Time observation finished: 10.44 a.m.

Total number of adults in setting: 2

Total number of children in setting: 20

First name(s) of child(ren) being observed: LUKE

Age(s): 4:4

Gender(s): M

Media used and justification (if necessary):

Supervisor's signature	Tutor's signature	Permission if applicable
C. Clarke	J. Brown.	✓

Child's initials: LF	Sex: M	Age: 4:4	Date and time Observed: 16.6.94	
ACTIVITY RECORD	LANGUAGE RECORD	TASK	SOCIAL	
1 min TC at activity table, making a model from junk.	TC → A "Pass the scissors." A → TC "When Jonah has finished"	Art	SG	
2 min TC waiting for scissors.	TC humming a song.	W	SG	
3 min TC cutting a large cereal box.	TC ←→ C (about the models they are making)	Art	SG	
4 min TC glueing model.	TC → A "Look at my aeroplane! Can I paint it?"	Art	SG	
5 min TC goes to paint table to paint his model.		Art	SOL	
6 min TC goes to bathroom to wash hands.	TC ←→ C (discussing Neighbours on TV) A watching	D A	PAIR +A	
7 min TC drying hands.	TC ←→ C (continue conversation) A leaves room	D A	PAIR	
8 min TC & C go outside & chase each other round playground.	shouting	I G	PAIR	

Codes : TC – Target Child   W – Waiting   IG – Informal games
         C – Child   Art – Art activities   SG – Small group
         A – Adult   D A – Domestic activities SOL – Solitary

OBSERVATION (TARGET CHILD): LUKE

INTERPRETATION

General comments
Luke has been in the nursery class almost a year. He is the eldest child, having a 2-year-old sister with cystic fibrosis and a 1-month-old baby brother. He attends regularly and has good health. His mother often stays with him and his siblings for an hour or so. She is always willing to help in any way she is able.

Evaluation
This type of observation was used by Kathy Sylva et al. for their research into concentration among pre-school children in Oxford, in 1980. The observation shows that Luke is a friendly and co-operative child, willing to wait his turn good-temperedly, and that he gets on well with peers and adults. He displays a number of manipulative and creative skills and shows maturity in wanting to finish his project. He shows independence in self care and is able to organise his activities without much adult direction. He is able to express his needs and converse socially with peers and adults.

Possible referral/course of action
Not applicable.

Personal learning
Luke's mother's time and attention is taken up with his brother and sister to a great extent, and I wondered if this affects Luke's behaviour in any way. This observation has shown me that he is coping well and he obviously feels safe and secure. I have learned that children can still thrive and develop, in spite of temporary difficult circumstances at home.

REFERENCE

Sylva K., Roy C. and Painter M., *Childwatching at Playgroup and Nursery School*, Grant McIntyre, 1980.

Child's initials: Sex: Age: Date and time Observed:			
ACTIVITY RECORD	LANGUAGE RECORD	TASK	SOCIAL
1 min			
2 min			
3 min			
4 min			
5 min			
6 min			
7 min			
8 min			

Time and event samples

TIME SAMPLES

Time samples are exactly that: a sample of time when you observe a child over a fairly long period. For example, you might choose to watch a child for one minute, from the time he or she arrives at the placement, at ten minute intervals, until home time. Preferably, you would try to do the samples at least once more in the same week. Children can show different behaviour early in the week, or early in the day, than they may do later on.

It is a good idea to attempt a time sample on a child about whom there is some concern. Before you start, describe the concern in some detail.

The following are examples of possible concerns:
- withdrawn behaviour
- shyness
- inability to relate to others (children or adults)
- crying constantly
- extreme lethargy
- extreme comfort behaviour (such as rocking, sucking, masturbating).

Ask your supervisor if there is a child he or she is concerned about and why. Observe the child closely for a day or so before starting the time sample. Write down in full all the problems the child seems to be facing. Completing the time sample will show you whether there is a real problem which needs intervention or referral, or whether, on the other hand, the concerns are not as worrying as was first thought.

Time samples may also be used to find out how children are using the toys and equipment in the placement. This is often helpful to the staff, who might think that all the equipment is being used equally, and then discover that some pieces of equipment are more popular than others. This could lead to enlarging or extending some areas of play.

EVENT SAMPLES

Event samples are used to record events during as long a period as possible, and at least for a week. The events you are looking out for are displays of aggressive behaviour. You would record these events each time they occurred, noting down the time of day, the duration of the event, whether they were provoked or not, and a comment on the seriousness of the behaviour. The aggressive behaviour might include:

- hitting and fighting
- biting
- spitting
- scratching
- extreme verbal abuse
- disruptive behaviour (such as destroying equipment or interfering with activities)
- acute loss of self control.

As in a time sample, try to observe the child first for a day or so, and then write down as fully as possible the perceived problem. You might find that the child only reacts when provoked by other children, or when he or she is tired or hungry. It is easy to presume that one child is the root cause of all disturbances. (Staff have been known to shout out a child's name at a fight and then discover that the child was absent that day.)

Time and event samples are used in placements to detect if children have a real behaviour problem or if it is just the perception of the staff. If the samples show that the child needs help, these sort of observations can be presented to professional colleagues. Sometimes these observations are used in case conferences where the future of the child is being discussed by a team of professional people. If the problem is not as serious as was first thought, the sample might show the staff that the way the child is being managed may be contributing in some way to the child's distress. The sample will enable the whole team to sit down together and see how the child can be helped in the placement to resolve a temporary anxiety.

ADVANTAGES OF TIME AND EVENT SAMPLES

- A collection of precise data
- More closely focused
- When completed, data is readily accessible
- Easily understood by other professionals and parent/carers
- Professional appearance and format.

DISADVANTAGES OF TIME AND EVENT SAMPLES

- Allocating the time to complete the task
- Remembering the time when doing time samples
- Keeping one child in sight at all times, without making it obvious to the child that he or she is being observed
- After first session, child may be absent for some time.

| 16 | Date: 6-6-94 | Method: TIME SAMPLE |

Aim and/or reason for observation: TO MONITOR &CONFIRM
ALICE'S WITHDRAWN BEHAVIOUR

Details of setting:

NURSERY CLASS

Immediate context:

N/A

Time observation started: 9.15 AM.

Time observation finished: 3.15 P.M. (FIRST OF A SERIES)

Total number of adults in setting: 3

Total number of children in setting: 26

First name(s) of child(ren) being observed: ALICE

Age(s): 4:1

Gender(s): F

Media used and justification (if necessary):

Supervisor's signature	Tutor's signature	Permission if applicable
G.C.Poole	K.Harris	✓

Time Sample

Concern: Heritage Language: ENGLISH

Alice is withdrawn from the nursery group. She only takes part in activities on her own. She does not join in story-time.

Time	Setting	Language	Social group
9.15	With mother in hall	Whimpering	2 - mother + Alice
9.35	Gazing out of window in book corner	None	Alone
9.55	Sucking thumb by climbing frame	None	Alone
10.15	Holding NN's hand. Outside play area	None - but listening to NN	2 - NN + Alice
10.35	Snack time. A at table with Gary (ch)	'I want my mummy' (addressed to Gary)	2 - Gary + Alice
10.55	Playing at water tray	None	Small group
11.15	Bathroom. Washing hands slowly	None	Alone
11.35	Story time. A sits with back to group	None	Isolated in large group
11.55	Dinner time. A eats voraciously	Asks for more	Small table, T and four children
12.15	Dinner time. A eating second pudding	None	As before
12.35	Outside play. A rides bike	'Look at me!' A to NN	Large group
12.55	As above.	Singing to herself	As above
1.15	Painting at easel	None	Alone
1.35	Sitting on NN's lap Thumb in mouth	Listening to NN	2 - NN + A
1.55	Lying on cushion in book corner. Sucking thumb	None	Alone
2.15	Asleep in book corner	None	Alone
2.35	Music session. A in home corner	Crying	2 - NN + A. NN tries to comfort A
2.55	Small world toys	Talking to herself	2 - Gary + A
3.15	Home time. Mother arrives	A bursts into tears. Hugs mother	2 - mother + A
		ch = child	A = Alice
		NN = Nursery nurse	T = teacher

OBSERVATION (TIME SAMPLE): ALICE

INTERPRETATION

General comments
Alice has been in the nursery group for nearly a year. At first, she settled quite happily, although she always had difficulty in separating from her mother.

Her grandmother, who lived with them, has been very ill recently and is in hospital. Alice has not been allowed to visit.

Evaluation
I decided to do a time sample as Jenny Laishley (1987) suggests using this method to observe closely children who display unhappiness. The time sample shows clearly that Alice is unhappy and, apart from the Nursery Nurse and one child, Gary, who lives next door to her, she does not wish to make relationships. The change in her behaviour is quite disturbing. In discussion with the Nursery Nurse, I have learned that her grandmother played a large part in Alice's early years, as her mother goes to work, and Alice is grieving for her.

Alice eats a great deal in the nursery, but is not overweight.

Possible referral/course of action
The Nursery Nurse is going to speak to Alice's mother and see if it is possible for her to visit her grandmother. She will try to persuade her to talk to Alice about her fears. She will also discuss Alice's enormous appetite, and try to assess if it is comfort eating or whether she is not getting enough to eat at home. It is always sensible to share concerns with parents and to work together to resolve problems, as described in the College Handout (1994).

Personal learning
From recording this time sample, I have learned that Alice is withdrawing herself more and more from groups of children and most adults. I have also learned that young children can grieve as fully as adults, as pointed out in the College Handout (1993).

REFERENCES

Laishley J., *Working with Young Children*, Edward Arnold, 1987.
College Handout, 'Working with parents', 1994.
College Handout, 'Bereavement', 1993.

Time Sample

Concern: Heritage Language:

Time	Setting	Language	Social group

You may photocopy this sheet for your own use. © Stanley Thornes (Publishers) Ltd 1994

| 24 | Date: 4/9/94 – 8/9/94 | Method: EVENT SAMPLE |

Aim and/or reason for observation:

GILLIAN BITES OTHER CHILDREN;
OCCASIONALLY KICKS & PUNCHES.

Details of setting:

WORKPLACE NURSERY

Immediate context:

N/A

Time observation started: CHILD OBSERVED FOR 1 WEEK.

Time observation finished:

Total number of adults in setting: 9

Total number of children in setting: 40

First name(s) of child(ren) being observed: GILLIAN

Age(s): 2:3

Gender(s): F

Media used and justification (if necessary):

Supervisor's signature	Tutor's signature	Permission if applicable
Kay Patel	G. Joseph.	✓

<u>Event Sample/Frequency Count</u>

<u>Concern:</u>
Gillian frequently bites both adults and children. She is aggressive and demanding.

Heritage Language: English

Day of week	No.	Duration	Provoked/Unprovoked	Comments on seriousness
Monday	1	2 secs.	U.P.	Gillian bit father as he left for work.
	2	1 min.	U.P.	Pushed Amit (1:9) over.
	3	2 secs.	U.P.	Bit Eric (2:3). Drew blood.
Tuesday	1	½ min.	U.P.	Hit Charley (3:0) with a wooden brick. Raised a bump on Charley's head.
	2	2 secs.	P.	Bit Charley (3:0) who pushed her over outside.
Wednesday	0			
Thursday	1	2 secs.	U.P.	Bit Amit (1:9). Not serious.
Friday	1	10 mins.	P.	Gillian's father arrived ½ an hour late. Gillian had a tantrum — inconsolable. She threw furniture around and attempted to bite nursery nurse.

OBSERVATION (EVENT SAMPLE): GILLIAN

INTERPRETATION

General comments
Gillian's mother has left the family group of father and two older siblings. Her father has a demanding job, but does his utmost to bring and collect Gillian on time. Gillian's language is immature, she has difficulty in expressing her needs through speech.

Evaluation
Jenny Laishley (1987) suggests using an event sample to show clearly how often an unhappy child takes out her feelings of anger and frustration on other children. Because Gillian's speech is poor, she often hits out rather than asking for what she wants. Biting is always a problem in a daycare group as the other parents, quite understandably, get angry when their child has been attacked. Therefore, it is important to try to deal with this as soon possible. This is described in the College Handout (1992).

Gillian's behaviour is worse at the beginning of the week, after a weekend at home. She becomes calmer as the week goes on, and in between the aggressive episodes is a happy and industrious child.

Possible referral/course of action
The placement organiser has made arrangements to see Gillian's father next Friday evening, when he has arranged to leave work early, to try to find out what Gillian's behaviour is like at home and how it is dealt with. It is important for the nursery and the family to work together. The speech therapist has been asked to come in and assess Gillian's language, as her inability to be understood is frustrating for her. Having two older brothers who understand her needs might make her less motivated to use words herself.

PERSONAL LEARNING

From closely observing Gillian this week I have learned that unhappiness can express itself in different ways in different children. I am going to discuss this observation at college, and I hope to get some suggestions as to how to stop Gillian from biting and attacking other children.

REFERENCES

Laishley J., *Working with Young Children*, Edward Arnold, 1987.
College Handout, 'The biter bit', 1992.

Event Sample/Frequency Count

Concern: Heritage Language:

Day of week	No.	Duration	Provoked/Unprovoked	Comments on seriousness

Taped language samples

To obtain an accurate sample of a child's speech, it is necessary to use a tape recorder in order to make sure that you have recorded everything the child has said. Before undertaking this task, you must obtain the permission of the placement and of the parent/carer. Make sure you are familiar with the mechanics of the recorder you are going to use. Remember to identify on tape brief details of the purpose of your recording, where you are and who you are with. The tape would then be included in your observation file, with or without a transcript. You will need to write an evaluation of the taped language. The tapes may be used for children who are thought to have a language delay or immature speech and can be very useful as an assessment tool for a speech therapist. They could be the basis on which to assess future progress.

Speech therapists often ask for help in recording the speech of very young children as the child may not be so confident and relaxed with a stranger.

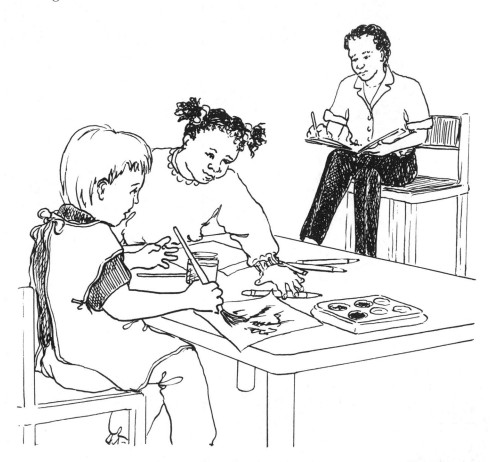

ADVANTAGES

- An accurate sample of speech is obtained
- Helpful to colleagues and other professionals
- Can be a key tool in referral
- Helps to integrate the theory of language development with the practice
- It can be helpful to play the speech sample to parent/carers, to initiate discussion.

DISADVANTAGES

- Difficulty in finding a tape recorder in good working order
- Requires certain technical skills to operate the recorder
- Doing the recording might put the child off, and inhibit language
- Background noise may interfere with the recording.

Sociograms

These are used either to indicate one particular child's social relationships within a group, or to look at friendship patterns of all the children within a group. Sometimes this highlights the unpopularity of a particular child and may well motivate the placement to help this child to establish fruitful relationships.

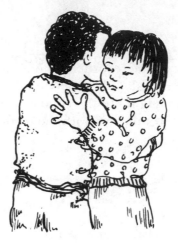

ADVANTAGES

- Can show quite clearly which children are most popular within the group
- Would indicate which children might need some help in establishing relationships with other children
- May make you more sensitive to changes in the social structure of the group.

DISADVANTAGES

- Relationships within the group may change from day to day
- Too much may be read into the data.

| 42 | Date: 4.5.94 | Method: Sociogram |

Aim and/or reason for observation:

To observe children's relationships with each other.

Details of setting:

Middle and top infant classroom

Immediate context:

—

Time observation started: 9.30 a.m.

Time observation finished: 12.30 p.m.

Total number of adults in setting: 2.

Total number of children in setting: 20 present (5 absent)

First name(s) of child(ren) being observed: as on graph

Age(s): 5:9 – 7:8

Gender(s): M & F

Media used and justification (if necessary):

Supervisor's signature	Tutor's signature	Permission if applicable
Jenny Bush	Angie Dixon.	✓

OBSERVATION (SOCIOGRAM): GROUP OF CHILDREN

INTERPRETATION

General comment
I asked the children to draw me a picture of their three best friends, and compiled the following graph to show the results. I only included those children in the class on the graph.

Evaluation
The graph shows that in general the children chose same-sex friends, with a few exceptions. The girls were more inclined to name a boy as a friend than the boys were a girl.

George (7:7), Victor (7:4) and Maz (7:7), who polled most votes, are amongst the oldest children in the class. Of these three, Maz's votes came entirely from boys. He is often in trouble at school because of his behaviour and can be quite aggressive, traits that make some of the boys look up to him and the girls avoid him.

Of the children who polled no votes, Rafik, Sara and Winston have only been in the class five weeks, having come up from Reception. Sara is a rather timid, often tearful girl who tends to stick close to Louise, who came from Reception with her, and was absent today. Winston chose his twin brother, Roger, and older sister, Emma, as his best friends. He is rather quiet, and tends to seek them out in the playground rather than join in with his classmates. Rafik nominated the three boys who were sitting at his table at the time. None of these three have established themselves in the class and would not be expected to have formed firm relationships within the group yet. Of the other two children who failed to get a vote, Danny (7:3) is again a quiet child who is frequently absent (as he was today), making it difficult to form relationships, and Sharon (7:8), who has quite marked behavioural problems, is often argumentative and aggressive. This would seem to show that such behaviour is seen as more acceptable in boys than in girls, even at this young age.

The children who chose each other tended to be amongst the older group, which is as expected as special friends tend to be made at 7 years, although I was surprised that this was more common amongst the boys. They tend to play and work together in a group, as is commonly seen at this age, but I would have expected to see more evidence of special friendships amongst the girls. Tara (7:5) proved most popular amongst the girls, but was absent today.

Most of the children seem to interact reasonably well together, although the few disruptive children can have an adverse effect on the whole group.

A Sociogram

	1	2	3	4	5	6	7	8	9	10
Edward	Aziz*	Mark								
George	Maz*	Billy	Nigel*	Rafik	Victor	Edward	Sharon	Catherine		
James	Victor									
Rafik										
Michelle	Sharon	Sara								
Nigel	Maz*	Billy*	Rafik							
Philippa	Mark*									
Catherine	James	Jyoti								
Sara										
Jyoti	George	Olive	Sharon							
Sharon										
Billy	Nigel*									
Mark	Aziz*	Trevor	Philippa*							
Maz	Nigel*	Rafik	James	George*	Edward					
Mary	James	Olive*								
Olive	Mary*									
Winston										
Aziz	Philippa	Mark*	Edward*							
Victor	Jyoti	Catherine	Aziz	Maz	Trevor*					
Trevor	Victor*	George								
(A) Peter	Billy	Trevor								
(A) Tara	Jyoti	Catherine	Philippa	Michelle						
(A) Tracey	Mary	Sara								
(A) Louise	Sara									
(A) Danny										

KEY

*	Mutual
(A)	Absent
▭	girls
▭	boys

POSSIBLE REFERRAL/COURSE OF ACTION

I have decided to repeat this sociogram in a month's time and, in particular, to monitor the progress of Danny and Sharon. I would expect Rafik, Sara and Winston to have made friends by this time.

Personal learning
I have learned that boys as well as girls make special friendships at this age, although Zick Rubin (1980) notes that such close relationships are more common in girls. I also found out that in this class aggressive behaviour is not so popular with the girls as it appears to be with the boys. I could not be certain if the boys really looked up to Maz or if they said that they liked him because they were somewhat afraid of him.

REFERENCE

Rubin Z., *Children's Friendships*, The Developing Child series, Fontana, 1980.

Movement and flow charts

Movement and flow charts are a shorthand way of presenting information about an individual or a group of children. A movement chart might be employed to see how a child uses the placement equipment by drawing a plan of the room and indicating by arrows the child's movement around the room.

ADVANTAGES

- Helpful in planning the use of equipment.

DISADVANTAGES

- Of limited use.

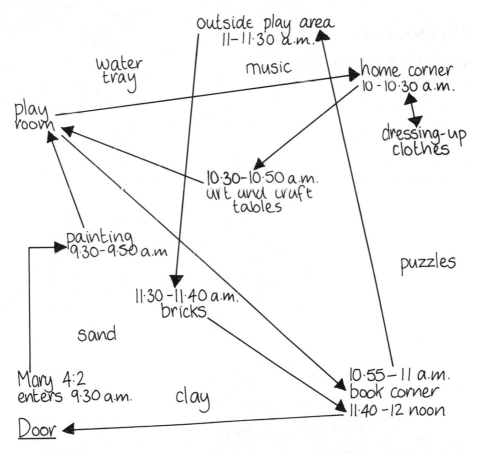

Example of a movement chart showing a 4-year-old child's use of activities during a pre-school morning session.

Graphs, pie and bar charts/histograms

These can be a useful way of collating information which you might find interesting about a group of children. For example, how do the children travel to school? How many of the children can skip? What is the most used piece of inside or outside equipment? Does the age of the child relate to his or her skill with a pair of scissors?

Sometimes these graphs and charts can be used in reports to managers and parent/carers, giving information about the placement in an easy to digest format. Parents can use pie charts at home, filling in a child's ability to acquire certain skills in order to share the information with the placement. Charts showing the use the children are making of the equipment provided might help staff to encourage children to use other types of equipment, perhaps putting out more stimulating material.

ADVANTAGES

- Quick and easy to collate
- Easy to read.

DISADVANTAGES

- Most charts only provide information about groups of children.
- They do not give much information about individuals.

Date: 25/1/94   Method: ⓐ PIE CHART
                          ⓑ BAR CHART

Aim and/or reason for observation:

TO OBSERVE A GROUP OF CHILDREN
SKIPPING AND DISPLAYING DIFFERING SKILLS.

Details of setting:

NURSERY CLASS

Immediate context:

OUTSIDE PLAY AREA

Time observation started: 9.30 a.m.

Time observation finished: 3.00 p.m.

Total number of adults in setting: 3

Total number of children in setting. 20

First name(s) of child(ren) being observed: —

Age(s): 3:2 ——— 4:9

Gender(s): M AND F

Media used and justification (if necessary):

Supervisor's signature   Tutor's signature   Permission if applicable

Kay Patel   Angie Dixon.   ✓

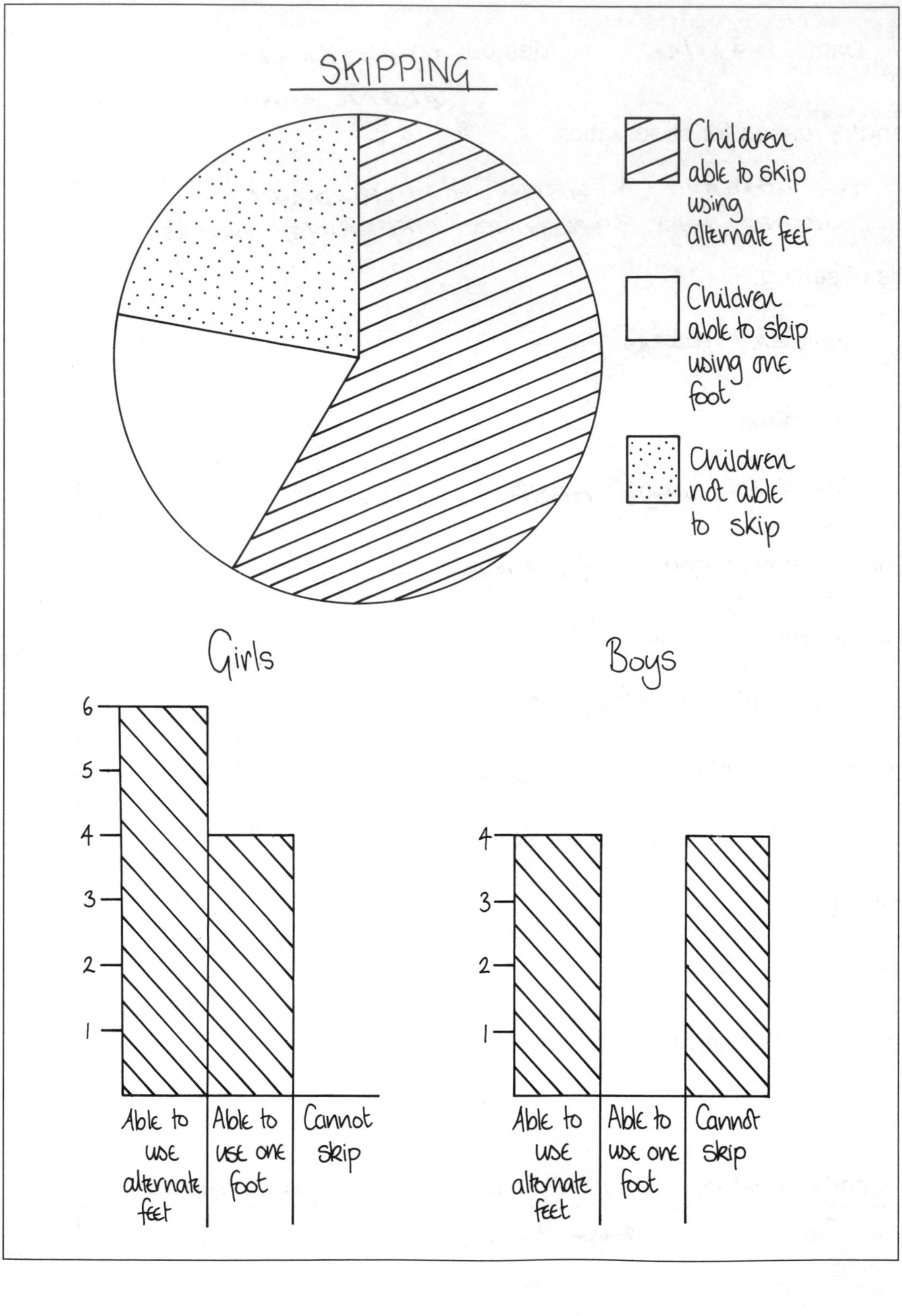
SKIPPING
Children able to skip using alternate feet
Children able to skip using one foot
Children not able to skip
Girls
Boys
6
5
4
3
2
1
Able to use alternate feet
Able to use one foot
Cannot skip
4
3
2
1
Able to use alternate feet
Able to use one foot
Cannot skip

OBSERVATION (PIE CHART/BAR CHART)

INTERPRETATION

General Comments
Over the course of one nursery day, I played a game with eighteen of the children in the nursery, which involved skipping skills where the children had to try to use alternate feet whilst crossing the playground.

Evaluation
As can be seen from the accompanying pie chart, more than half the children in the class can skip using alternate feet. This majority is made up of the older children (the rising fives and the 4-year-olds). Mary Sheridan (1991) states that this skill is usually found in the 5-year-old child. Of the remaining children, half cannot skip at all and the rest only on one foot. Of the children who cannot skip at all, only one is a 4-year-old, and all the rest are 3-year-old. This is age appropriate as 3-year-olds do not have the muscle control to co-ordinate this activity. The bar chart shows that more girls than boys can skip using alternate feet, and that none of the girls are unable to skip at all. The four boys who cannot skip are the youngest in the class.

Possible referral/course of action
Not applicable.

PERSONAL LEARNING

I found out that the skipping skills in the class closely follow developmental theory.

REFERENCES

Sheridan M., *Children's Developmental Progress from Birth to Five Years*, NFER, 1991.

31	Date: 28.3.94 Method: HISTOGRAM

Aim and/or reason for observation:

To observe the reading ability of a group of children.

Details of setting:

Infant school

Immediate context:

Corridor — small library area

Time observation started: 9.30 a.m.

Time observation finished: 3.25 p.m.

Total number of adults in setting: 2.

Total number of children in setting: 25.

First name(s) of child(ren) being observed: ——

Age(s): 6.1 — 6.9

Gender(s): M & F

Media used and justification (if necessary):

Supervisor's signature	Tutor's signature	Permission if applicable
C. Power.	1. Ded.	✓

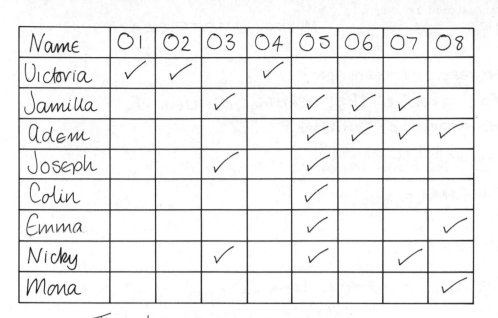

Name	01	02	03	04	05	06	07	08
Victoria	✓	✓		✓				
Jamilla			✓		✓	✓	✓	
Adem					✓	✓	✓	✓
Joseph			✓		✓			
Colin					✓			
Emma					✓			✓
Nicky			✓		✓		✓	
Mona								✓

Tick list to show individual reading ability on the day

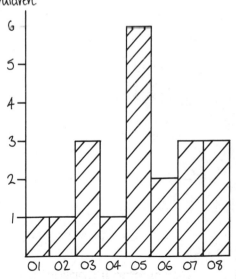

no of children

Key
01 Read in true sense
02 Recognise all 3 letter words
03 Recognise some 3 letter words
04 Recognise all 2 letter words
05 Recognise some 2 letter words
06 Read book from memory
07 Used pictures as prompts
08 Showed no interest

INDIVIDUAL REPORTS IN BRIEF

Time: 09.50   Name: Jamilla
Jamilla picked out four books from the basket. The first book, *Round and Round*, was read through quickly. But this was done through memory rather than reading in the true sense. The second book, *Doctors and Nurses*, was more of a challenge. The story was not a familiar one to Jamilla. Some two- and three-letter words were recognised, but Jamilla found it very hard going.

Jamilla used some of the pictures that accompanied the text to work out what was written, and tried very hard.

With the third book, *The Storm*, she was back on familiar ground and read it from memory. Jamilla made a very brave attempt at the last book, *The Pumpkin*, using pictures and recognised words to work out the story. Most of the story line was missed, but Jamilla still did well.

Time: 10.00   Name: Adem
Goldilocks and the Three Bears was Adem's choice from the book basket. This version is a very hard book to read for this age band. Adem picked out this book and started to tell the story from memory of a different version of the story. When stopped, Adem tried to read the book, but was only able to recognise some two- and three-letter words. Adem never really showed any interest in reading today and spent his time looking around.

Time: 10.05   Name: Joseph
Joseph also chose *Goldilocks* as his book. He started enthusiastically enough, but lost interest when he realised that the book was too hard for him. Again, Joseph realised some two- and three-letter words. When offered a second choice of book, Joseph declined and his concentration drifted further away.

Time: 10.15   Name: Colin
Colin was only interested for a very short while. He managed to recognise very few words in the two-letter bracket. After two pages, he started to wander around the corridor, so he was taken back to class.

Time: 10.18   Name: Emma
Emma chose two books, *The Pumpkin* and *Plop*. She started with *Plop*. Emma sat on her hands, legs swinging back and forth. Her attention was never really focused on the books and she showed no real interest. However, Emma did recognise some two-letter words.

Time: 15.10   Name: Nicky
Nicky struggled with the books that he chose. These were *The storm* and *Round and Round*. He was able to recognise some two- and three-letter words and tried very hard.

Time: 15.15   Name: Mona
Mona didn't want to read at all and appeared too upset when asked to do so. So this was abandoned.

Time: 15.16   Name: Victoria
Victoria picked two books, *The cat, the bird and the tree* and *Animals*. Victoria sailed through these books with ease, pointing to each individual word as she spoke them. On first impressions, I thought that this was done by pure memory. But when checked by asking what other words were, it was evident that Victoria can actually read in the true sense. She was only stopped by a few words, for example 'Redbreast' (as in robin) and 'afraid'.

Victoria enjoys reading and was upset when asked to stop as home time loomed closer.

OBSERVATION (HISTOGRAM)

INTERPRETATION

General Comments

This observation follows a request from the class teacher to take a group of children for reading practice. The children and the books were selected by the teacher, and I took the children one by one out into the corridor. The results were first recorded on a tick list and a brief written report was made for each child. A histogram was added later.

Evaluation

As can be seen from the histogram and the tick list, there is only one child in this group of 6-year-olds who can read fluently. The reports showed that, although there is some variation in ability, there is only real concern about one child, Colin. Some writers, such as Henry Pluckrose (1970) have pointed out that this need not be a cause for concern, as long as the child is attaining well in other areas, for example numeracy and social relationships.

The concentration time span varied but this may be due to the time of day when more interesting activities were going on in the classroom.

Possible referral/course of action

With the teacher's permission, I would like to do a follow-up activity with the same children in a month's time, at a different time of day. I have realised how much opportunity for reading most children need, and that reading is taught and not caught! I will spend some time each day with Colin to build a relationship and, hopefully, he will then be able to relax more with me.

PERSONAL LEARNING

I learned how difficult it is to assess in one session children's ability in any learning situation. One has to take into account that the children do not know me very well, we were out in the noisy corridor, interesting activities were happening in the classroom and three of the children appear very tired at this time of day. This has demonstrated to me the strong distractions that hamper a child's concentration, as highlighted in the College Handout (1992).

REFERENCES

Pluckrose H., *Children in their Primary Schools*, Harper & Row, 1980.
College Handout, 'Becoming a reader', 1992.

Checklist

Checklists or developmental guides are often used for assessing a child on one particular day, but can be used over a longer period. The placement might decide to do a 'snapshot' observation of all children within six weeks of entry to a nursery placement, or it might be used for a child about whom there is some concern. Checklists can also be used for all the children in the placement on a regular basis to enable the staff to plan for each child's needs.

They can be specific, looking at one area of development or assessing a child's behaviour, or they can be more general, covering all areas. There are some frequently used charts. Many placements will adapt or devise their own checklist. As an example, educational psychologist Hannah Mortimer has published a booklet containing twenty-one 'playladders'. These are checklists of young children's activities in a variety of settings. They are a method of recording how a child plays at present, and provide ideas on helping the child to reach the next stage.

You should have a good knowledge of the child before you attempt a checklist. Results may otherwise be distorted by the impact of an unfamiliar adult.

Activity
Using your library, find as many developmental guides, checklists and assessment schedules, as you can.
Which professionals use checklists? In what establishments?

Checklists often highlight areas of a child's development that have previously gone unnoticed. For example, a child who appears physically very competent sometimes has difficulty in controlling wheeled toys. Being aware of this, the staff are then able to provide practice and encouragement. A child can also be shown to be mature in some way and this can be supported and extended.

After completing any checklist, you will need to write a summary, showing what you have learned and suggesting any possible course of action the placement might take to help or encourage the child.

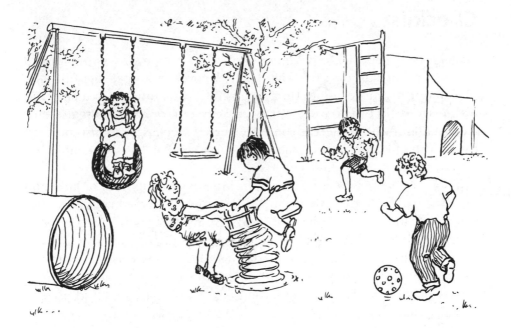

ADVANTAGES

- A quick way of presenting a great deal of information
- Results are obvious and readily understandable
- Can be useful to combine with a longitudinal observation when carrying out a child study
- The same guide can be used for several children to find out more about the group. This can indicate gender differences or show that there are none
- Can be used by parent/carers.

DISADVANTAGES

- Care must be taken to maintain objectivity. It is tempting to put a tick against skills which you previously thought the child had achieved.
- Checklists may not give a true picture if the child is less than co-operative on the day, or if the child is unwell.
- The child should be unaware of being assessed or may become stressed. You will have to show ingenuity to turn the assessment into a game as otherwise the data will be invalid and unreliable.

Hannah Mortimer
Educational Psychologist
North Yorkshire L.E.A.

'Playladders' can be obtained by sending a cheque for £1.50 to Hannah Mortimer, Ainderby Hall, Northallerton, North Yorkshire DL7 9QJ. Parts of the booklet are illustrated in this handout.

PLAYLADDERS

Playladders are checklists of young children's play as they go about their activities in nursery, playgroup or at home. They are a method of observing and recording how a child plays now, and they provide ideas on how to help the child reach the next step. 'Playladders' combine the step-by-step approach developed in special education, with the practicalities of what goes on in a busy playroom.

The Playladders booklet contains 21 playladders, each one representing an activity typically available for under fives, for example: climbing frames, painting, home corner, book corner or glue table. Each activity is broken down into progressive steps and skills. The emphasis is on flexibility, and users are encouraged to adapt, modify or add to the ladders to suit the particular child, culture and setting. There are also blank playladders to build up for yourself.

Playladders were originally designed for nursery and playgroup staff who had children with special educational needs in their classes.

Playladders provide the ideas for moving one step at a time from simple to more complex play, encouraging young children in their learning.

AN EXAMPLE OF THE PLAYLADDERS IN USE

Beth was a three-year-old who had just started at her local nursery class. At first, she was very quiet and spent the entire session walking up and down the room pushing a trolley. She resisted any advances from the adults and children. We used the Playladders to map her play; this needed a lot of help from her mother as Beth did so little for us in nursery. Together we concluded that Beth was still at an early stage in all areas of her play and social life, and that pushing a trolley was her safest option in her new and unfamiliar setting.

One of us began to befriend Beth, who gradually allowed the contact. She began to seek this helper out and would park her trolley for a moment while watching other children play, so long as the helper was nearby. She would help to clear up using her trolley and, in time, park it long enough to draw a scribble which she then carried around in it. Using the Playladders for ideas, and the trolley as a starting point, Beth gradually increased her repertoire of play and felt safe to leave her trolley and join in.

POSTSCRIPT

If you don't work in a playgroup, but in some other kind of setting, don't be tempted to dismiss this format out of hand. It can readily be adapted for other settings. For example, during the trialling of the pack, this format was developed by a junior school teacher into a complete record-keeping system for children's progress in physical education.

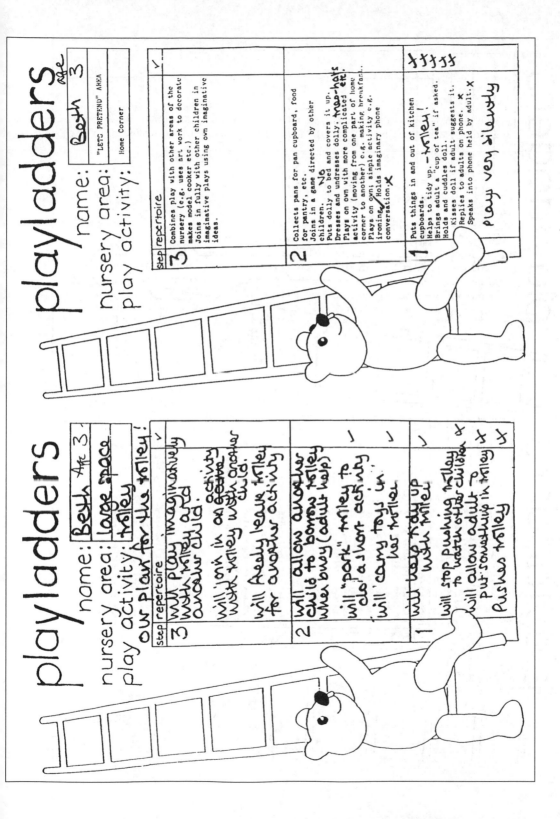

playladders

name: Beth Age 3
nursery area: "LETS PRETEND" AREA
play activity: Home Corner

step	repertoire	✓
3	Combines play with other areas of the nursery (e.g. uses art work to decorate makes model cooker etc.) Joins in fully with other children in imaginative plays using own imaginative ideas.	✓
2	Collects pans for pan cupboard, food for pantry, etc. Joins in a game directed by other children. No Puts dolly to bed and covers it up. two-hats Dresses and undresses dolly. Plays on own with more complicated etc. activity (moving from one part of home corner to another) e.g. making breakfast. Plays on own: simple activity e.g. ironing. Holds imaginary phone conversation. X	
1	Puts things in and out of kitchen cupboards. Helps to tidy up. — trolley! Brings adult a "cup of tea" if asked. Holds and cuddles doll. Kisses doll if adult suggests it. X Replies to adults on phone. X Speaks into phone held by adult. X	plays very silently ↑↑↑↑↑

playladders

name: Beth Age 3
nursery area: large space
play activity: trolley
our play for the trolley!

step	repertoire	✓
3	Will play imaginatively with trolley and another child. Will join in an activity with trolley with another child. Will freely leave trolley for another activity.	✓
2	Will allow another child to borrow trolley when busy (adult help). Will "park" trolley to do a short activity. Will carry toys in her trolley.	✓ ✓
1	Will help tidy up with trolley. Will stop pushing trolley to watch other children. Will allow adult to put something in trolley. Pushes trolley.	✓ ✓ ✓ ✓

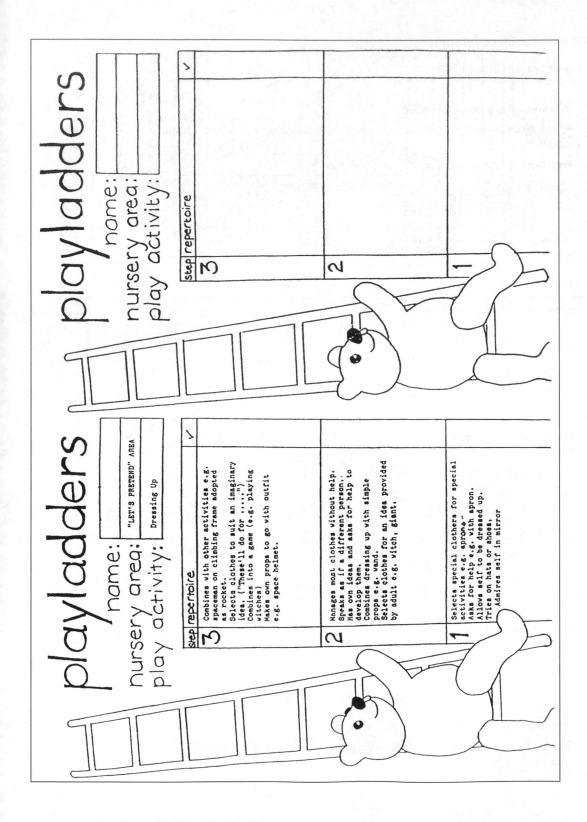

playladders

name:
nursery area:
play activity:

step	repertoire	✓
3		
2		
1		

playladders

name:
nursery area: "LET'S PRETEND" AREA
play activity: Dressing Up

step	repertoire	✓
3	Combines with other activities e.g. spaceman on climbing frame adopted as rocket. Selects clothes to suit an imaginary idea. ("These'll do for .....") Combines into a game (e.g. playing witches) Makes own props to go with outfit e.g. space helmet.	
2	Manages most clothes without help. Speaks as if a different person. Has own ideas and asks for help to develop them. Combines dressing up with simple props e.g. wand. Selects clothes for an idea provided by adult e.g. witch, giant.	
1	Selects special clothes for special activities e.g. apron. Asks for help e.g. with apron. Allows self to be dressed up. Tries on hats or shoes. Admires self in mirror	

Children's social development

I. Individual Attributes: The child	Yes	No
1. Is **usually** in a positive mood		
2. Is not **excessively** dependent on the teacher, Nursery Nurse or other adults		
3. **Usually** comes to the nursery or school willingly		
4. **Usually** copes with rebuffs and reverses adequately		
5. Shows the capacity to empathise		
6. Has positive relationship with one or two peers; shows capacity to really care about them, miss them if absent, etc.		
7. Displays the capacity for humour		
8. Does not seem to be acutely or chronically lonely		
II. Social Skill Attributes: The child usually		
1. Approaches the others positively		
2. Expresses wishes and preferences clearly; gives reasons for actions and positions		
3. Asserts own rights and needs appropriately		
4. Is not easily intimidated by bullies		
5. Expresses frustration and anger effectively and without harming others or property		
6. Gains access to ongoing groups at play and work		
7. Enters ongoing discussion on the subject; makes relevant contributions to ongoing activities		
8. Takes turns fairly easily		
9. Shows interest in others; exchanges information with and requests information from others appropriately		
10. Negotiates and compromises with others appropriately		
11. Does not draw inappropriate attention to self		
12. Accepts and enjoys peers and adults of ethnic groups other than his or her own		
13. Interacts non-verbally with other children with smiles, waves, nods, etc.		
III. Peer Relationship Attributes: The child is		
1. **Usually** accepted versus neglected or rejected by other children		
2. **Sometimes** invited by other children to join them in play, friendship, and work		

D.E. McClellan and L.G. Katz 1992

SHEFFIELD LEA

An Admission Profile

Completion of the profile

It is envisaged that the format can be adapted to meet the specific needs of individual teachers and schools.

The profile is intended to give a general picture of the child and will highlight areas of concern for further work. Teachers will find that the profile does not take very long to complete, particularly as staff become more confident with the range of behaviours illustrated.

From the range of behaviours 1–5 under each sub-heading, choose the number which most clearly represents the stage at which the child is operating. This number should be written on the profile summary grid which follows the section. This profile summary can be completed during the first six weeks after entry and will give a broad overall picture of the child which can be discussed with colleagues, parents and support staff. This profile precedes the developmental record for children in nursery schools and classes.

It is suggested that the profile be completed at the end of the child's settling-in period in school when the staff are aware of the child's behaviour and development in a wide range of activities. A return to this profile at regular intervals would enable staff to monitor the child's progress.

Name ....

Date of birth

Admission date

Attendance

Anything particular relating to all-round development

Physical development

Gross motor skills	
Excellent co-ordination and control, e.g. running, climbing, balancing, throwing, kicking	1
Usually well co-ordinated	2
Satisfactory	3
Below average, tends to be awkward	4
Very poorly co-ordinated, clumsy, often falls over, bumps into things	5

Fine motor skills	
Excellent manipulation of pencils, small construction materials	1
Above average control and co-ordination	2
Satisfactory	3
Awkward in fine control and manipulation	4
Very poor fine co-ordination and manipulative skills, great difficulties in holding small tools	5

Social and emotional development

Co-operation	
Very keen to work/play with others	1
Enjoys working/playing with others	2
Satisfactory	3
Prefers to work/play on own most of time	4
Never (or rarely) works/plays with others	5

Temperament	
Even tempered, nearly always happy and in control of self. Can adapt to new situations, shows initiative, independence	1
Generally happy and controlled, adapts easily and with self confidence	2
Satisfactory	3
Can be irritable and moody in new situations	4
Finds new situations very disturbing, becomes excitable, withdrawn or loses control	5

Acceptance by peers	
Very popular	1
Well accepted member of the group	2
Satisfactory	3
On fringe of peer group; peers tend to shun him/her	4
Disliked and rejected by peers	5

Attitudes to peers	
Very considerate and thoughtful to others	1
Usually kind and considerate	2
Satisfactory	3
Often wary; can be aggressive in response to others. Tends to avoid other children	4
Always or nearly always disregards others' feelings	5

Attitudes to adults	
Nearly always keen to please, to do well	1
Helpful and co-operative most of the time	2
Satisfactory	3
Can be unco-operative and unresponsive; disruptive on occasions	4
Often refuses to co-operate, can be very disruptive	5

General development and attitude to learning

Degree of involvement in task	
Excellent attention to task, works well and is not affected by general classroom activity	1
Above average attention to task, only occasionally distracted	2
Satisfactory	3
Below average, tends to look around, gets distracted	4
Very poor ability to attend to one task, highly distracted by noise or movement	5

Concentration and ability to organise	
Nearly always concentrates until concluded. Very good ability to organise self	1
Generally concentrates well	2
Satisfactory	3
Attention span limited; problems with organising	4
Very short attention span, tasks usually unfinished, very disorganised	5

Motivation	
Very keen to learn, always or nearly always interested in learning tasks	1
Above average eagerness to learn	2
Satisfactory	3
Below average, tends to want to avoid learning situations	4
Apathetic and uninterested, difficult to motivate	5

Level of concern felt	
Excellent general development, causes no concern	1
General development is very good	2
Satisfactory	3
Some concern about general development, overall below average	4
General concern about development, overall development is slow	5

Summary of profile

Score		1	2	3	4	5
PHYSICAL DEVELOPMENT	Gross motor skills					
	Fine motor skills					
SOCIAL AND EMOTIONAL DEVELOPMENT	Co-operation					
	Attitudes to peers					
	Acceptance by peers					
	Temperament					
	Attitudes to adults					
GENERAL DEVELOPMENT AND ATTITUDES TO LEARNING	Motivation					
	Concentration and ability to organise					
	Degree of involvement in task					
	Level of concern felt					

ANY ACTION NEEDED	

Photographs and video recordings

These should be used rarely and only with the permission of the parent/carer and the placement. They should only be used to demonstrate a skill, in the same way that you might include a child's drawing if you wanted to illustrate his or her competence at an activity. They can be useful in a longitudinal study, to demonstrate, for example, locomotive skills.

Photographs and video recordings must be evaluated and commented upon. 'Pretty' photographs have no place in a professional file.

ADVANTAGES

- Statement that should stand up on its own
- Less writing involved.

DISADVANTAGES

- What you see may not be obvious to other people
- Usually need to obtain permission
- Children can be recognised at a later date.

Some other forms of assessment

THE HIGH/SCOPE TECHNIQUE

There are numerous ways of assessing children, using all types of tests and charts. High/Scope uses an ongoing type of assessment, noting progress in development of each child over a three-month period.

High/Scope Preschool Key Experiences

Creative Representation

- Recognizing objects by sight, sound, touch, taste, and smell
- Imitating actions and sounds
- Relating pictures, photographs, and models to real places and things
- Pretending and role-playing
- Making models out of clay, blocks, etc.
- Drawing and painting

Language and Literacy

- Talking with other about personally meaningful experiences
- Describing objects, events, and relations
- Having fun with language: Listening to stories and poems, making up stories and rhymes
- Writing in various ways: drawing, scribbling, letter-like forms, invented spelling, conventional forms
- Reading in various ways: reading storybooks, signs, symbols and other print materials

Social Relations/Initiative

- Making and expressing choices, plans and decisions
- Solving problems encountered in play
- Taking care of one's own needs
- Expressing feelings in words
- Participating in group routines
- Being sensitive to the feelings, interests, and needs of others
- Building relationships with children and adults
- Creating and experiencing collaborative play
- Dealing with social conflict in constructive ways

Movement

- Moving in place
- Moving from place to place
- Moving with objects
- Describing movement
- Interpreting movement directions
- Expressing creativity in movement
- Feeling and expressing beat
- Moving with others to a common beat

Music

- Responding to music
- Making and describing sounds
- Playing musical instruments
- Singing

Classification

- Exploring and describing similarities, differences and the attributes of things
- Sorting and matching
- Using and describing something in several different ways
- Distinguishing between "some" and "all"
- Holding more than one attribute in mind at a time
- Describing characteristics something does not possess or what class it does not belong to

Seriation

- Comparing attributes: longer/shorter; rougher/smoother, etc.
- Arranging several things one after another in a series or pattern and describing the relationships: big, bigger, biggest
- Fitting one ordered set of objects to another through trial and error

Number

- Comparing number and amount to determine "more", "less", "fewer", "same amount"

- Arranging two sets of objects in one-to-one correspondence
- Counting objects as well as counting by rote

Space

- Filling and emptying
- Fitting things together and taking them apart
- Changing the shape and arrangement of objects (folding, twisting, stretching, stacking)
- Observing things and places from different spatial viewpoints
- Experiencing and describing relative positions, directions and distances of things in the immediate environment (play space, building, neighbourhood)
- Interpreting spatial relations in drawings, pictures, and photographs

Time

- Starting and stopping an action on signal
- Experiencing and describing different rates of movement
- Experiencing and comparing time intervals
- Experiencing and anticipating change and sequences of events.

HIGH/SCOPE EDUCATIONAL RESEARCH FOUNDATION

Pam Lafferty 1992

High/Scope Endorsed Trainer   Child Anecdotal Record (C.A.R.)   (Condensed Sheet)

Child's Name: Jinnie   Birth Date: 16/9/86   (Remember to date all entries)

LANGUAGE AND LITERACY	CREATIVE REPRESENTATION	CLASSIFICATION	SERIATION	NUMBER
5/9/91:- J was sitting looking at a story book and telling a story from the pictures	2/9/91:- Playing with the plastic animals and making the appropriate sounds for horse, cow and pig	7/10/91:- Stacked up the brick piles into separate colours - red, blue, green and yellow	11/91:- Remarked that the new fruit bowl was heavier than the old one	18/9/91:- Said "a few means not a lot"
3/9/91:- Said "Go Jo Flow Blow - they sound the same"	24/9/91:- Nailed two pieces of wood together in a cross shape and said it was an aeroplane	12/11/91:- Said "My boots are red and yours are blue"	27/9/91:- Comparing paint brushes said "Mine's larger and fatter that yours"	18/11/91:- Cut dough into four pieces and said "I've made four cakes"
3/12/91:- Whilst sitting on a toilet seat said that she was sitting on an "O"	8/11/91:- Drew a robin with minute details and coloured it in accurately with red	6/12/91:- Looking at the words "Jack" and "Jake" said that the two names were nearly the same, just a little bit different	17/12/91:- Chose a number of triangle shapes from the box and arranged them in order of increasing size	6/12/91:- Counted 7 penguins accurately on a friend's jumper

SPACE	TIME	MUSIC AND MOVEMENT	SOCIAL RELATIONS/INITIATIVE
23/9/91:- Talking to another child about a hat said "You need the ribbons at the back, not the side"	8/10/91:- When the tidy-up sound was made, J began to put things from the floor into their correct basket	12/9/91:- Was walking around the nursery on all fours swaying from side to side being and elephant	4/10/91:- On coming from the garden to the inside, stopped in the doorway to leave muddy wellingtons outside
30/10/91:- Folded a piece of card in half to form a tunnel and then walked plastic animals through it and used the word through	28/11/91:- Said "If you want to find me later, I'll be in the Book Area"	21/10/91:- For the first time managed to use her legs to make the swing go	29/10/91:- Took a friend into the bathroom and used a cotton wool ball to wipe mud from his knee
9/12/91:- Noticed a triangular patch of light on the carpet and found a triangle shape to fit exactly on top of it	29/11/91:- Looked at a list of names on the board and said "It will be Matthew's turn to open the door tomorrow"	13/12/91:- Used scissors to cut a "fringe" along the side of a piece of paper	12/12/91:- At snack time said "G only likes bananas - please save one for him"

Child's Name:

Remember to date all entries

Language and literacy	Creative representation	Classification	Seriation ordering	Space	Number	Time	Movement and music	Soc/Relations Initiative

For more information about High/Scope Curriculum and key experiences contact High/Scope UK, Copperfield House, 190–192 Maple Road, Penge, London SE20 8HT. Tel. 081 676 0220

THE PIAGET CONSERVATION TEST

A test you might like to carry out in your 4- to 7-year-old placement is a Piaget conservation test. These are ways of testing mathematical concepts in young children and quite often have revelationary results. You must be careful to be very neutral and objective when using these.

CONSERVATION TESTS

According to Piaget, children of 5 or 6 years of age cannot conserve. This means that their thought processes are dominated by the appearances of things, and they do not realise that the volume of an object may not change just because the appearance changes.

Conservation occurs when children are able to take in several features of the objects they are looking at all at the same time. You must be neutral when administering these tests and be sure to praise the child whatever the answer.

Conservation of number

Show a child two rows of buttons, and ask him or her to count each row. When he or she has agreed that there is the same number in both rows, spread one row of buttons out. Then ask if either of the two rows contains more buttons. A child who cannot conserve will say that the spread out row must have more buttons.

Conservation of mass

Show the child two balls of clay and get his or her agreement that both balls contain the same amount of clay. Then roll one of the balls into a sausage shape and ask the child if they still contain the same amount of clay. A child who cannot conserve will say that the sausage shape must contain more than the other ball, as it looks as if it contains more.

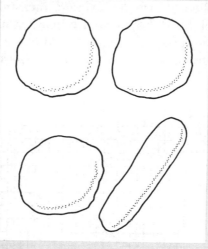

Conservation of volume

Ask the child to pour water into two identical tall thin jars until the child is satisfied that both contain an equal amount. Then, in front of the child, pour the water from one of the jars into a shorter but wider jug. A child who cannot conserve will say the tall jar contains more liquid.

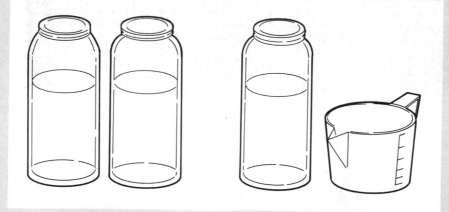

PERCENTILE CHARTS

Percentile charts are used for recording the weight, height and head circumference of babies and children. There are separate charts for boys and girls.

The charts were compiled after taking the measurements of thousands of children.

The thick line labelled 50th is the average measurement. The line marked 97th shows weights of boys who are heaviest in their group. As you record a measurement regularly on a chart the line will show you the child's individual progress, and allow you to compare that child with other children.

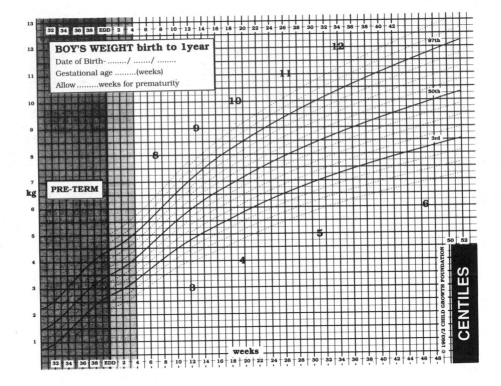

Range of observations

Your tutors will indicate to you the requirements of your particular course.

Once you start building up a file of observations, you must be careful to include a full range. All observations need to be child-centred, and focused on the child or children. Adults will often figure in your observations, but it is the reaction of the child to the adult that you need to note.

You will need to:

1 Demonstrate that you have covered every area of child development (physical, cognitive, language, social, emotional and moral), while some observations, such as your child study, examine the development of the whole child .

2 Cover a range of learning situations, activities, routines and experiences, reflecting the importance of play and language in children's lives and development. Make sure you demonstrate a variety of play situations, such as solo play, messy play, parallel play, group play, creative play, imaginative play and so on. Language and interaction should be observed between child and adult, and child to child, showing both reported speech, understanding and social interaction, such as you might observe during the routine of story time.

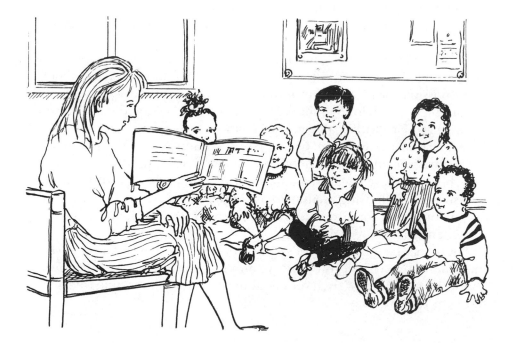

3 Cover a range of types and patterns of behaviour, to include an emotional range from withdrawn behaviour to aggressive disruptive behaviour. Make sure you include the full spectrum, and do not just concentrate on extremes.

4 Observe all the age ranges (0 to 1, 1 to 4, and 4 to 7 years). Half the observations should relate to the 1 to 4 age group, with whom you will be spending most of your time.

5 Ensure that you complete observations in all your placements.

6 Show aspects of physical care and routines, such as washing, feeding, dealing with accidents, caring for the sick child, toilet training etc., and health routines such us screening and surveillance, immunisation, and so on.

7 Cover situations indoor and outdoor in the placement.

8 Cover some situations that occur outside the placement. You will need to have permission from the adult responsible for the child, who should sign the observation and include their name and address. Your tutor should countersign the observation. This obviously raises issues of confidentiality, and may restrict the number that you include.

9 Cover large and small groups and the individual child. A quarter of observations should relate to children in groups.

10 Cover children's learning and development within the context of the National Curriculum, showing the growth of early literacy, numeracy and scientific understanding.

11 Include some children with particular needs, such as distressed children, gifted children and children with special educational needs.

12 Cover major events and transitions in children's lives, such as settling into nursery school, birth of a sibling, loss of a parent, etc.

13 If possible, observe children whose first language is not English, and attempt to include children from a wide a range of different backgrounds within all your placements.

14 Use as many different types of observations as you can, such as naturalistic observations of free activity; structured observations where you have organised an activity to gain particular information; 'snapshots' showing an immediate impression of a child at one point in time; and longitudinal studies, recording information over an extended period of time.

There may be other areas of special interest to you, or relating to your placement, that you wish to observe and record. If you have any doubts about the suitability of such observations, it would be sensible to discuss this with your tutor.

Progression of skills

Completion of a file of observations will allow you to become a professional expert at observation techniques, and you will be much valued for this skill in many multi-disciplinary teams. It is by no means an easy skill to develop and you may take quite a while before you feel really comfortable in demonstrating your techniques. Your college will devote time each week to help you gain confidence and your placement will allow you adequate time to practise your skills. In building up your file during your course you will progress from simple structured written records of one child over a short period of time to complex techniques observing groups of children over several weeks. Your increasing skills will be demonstrated in your file and will be acknowledged by the external moderators to the course.

Self appraisal

From time to time you might find it useful to look at your observations and assess them for yourself. Having carried out this task, it is occasionally a good idea to check your self-appraisal with that of your tutor and your supervisor. You may find, on rare occasions, that they disagree with each other on your progress and perhaps you could ask them to discuss this during a visit to the placement.

One way of grading this could be to give yourself a mark of 5 for excellence, 4 for very good, 3 for satisfactory, 2 for could do better and 1 for unsatisfactory.

Having completed the appraisal, you may be able to identify the areas where you need to seek help in order to progress. In discussion with your tutor you may develop an action plan together. For example, if you have difficulty in using one particular method of recording, your supervisor might be able to write an observation with you, using this technique. If your observations are considered too messy, you might be able to arrange access to a word processor. If interpretation is the problem, your tutor could guide you towards further reading.

Self-appraisal checklist

Date: _____

	You	Your tutor	Your supervisor
Number of observations			
Range across the areas of development			
Range across the age groups			
Range of techniques			
Choosing appropriate observations			
Presented in a professional manner			
Awareness of strict confidentiality			
Making progress in interpreting observations			
Working systematically – setting aside time each week			
Seeking help in difficulty			
Accepting and acting on constructive criticism			

Questions to ask yourself:
Are you up-to-date?

Are you finding the process is becoming easier?

What areas do you find easy?

What areas do you find difficult?

You may photocopy this sheet for your own use. © Stanley Thornes (Publishers) Ltd 1994

5 HOW TO USE YOUR OBSERVATIONS

This chapter covers:
- **In the college**
- **In the placement**
- **Objectivity**
- **Sharing information**
- **Compiling a file**
- **Presentation**
- **References/Bibliography**
- **Using your observations in your future professional role**

In the college

As soon as you have finished your first observation and it has been signed in the placement as a true record, you will hand it to your tutor to read, sign and comment on. This should be a regular process, so that you are observing children routinely. It is easier for supervisors and tutors to comment and help you if the observations are presented systematically, in small numbers, after each placement week. Observations given to your supervisor months after the event may well be forgotten and your supervisor might be reluctant to sign them. Tutors like to see work every time you come back to college so that they can pick up on any problems you might be having with the children or in the placement generally.

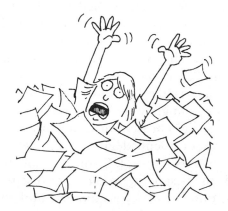

Many colleges use observations to form the basis of group discussion. You will read out your observation, and the group will have a chance to comment on it and help you, perhaps with your interpretation. Your tutor will make sure that you are all on the right path in your interpretations and a great deal will be learned about good practice, individual behaviour and developmental norms. This is an excellent way of integrating theory with practice.

As you progress, your tutor will use some of this time to explain different techniques and methods of recording information. At times, the group will be encouraged to use a particular technique, so that you will obtain immediate feedback in college. Your longitudinal studies will need to be carefully monitored, probably on a one-to-one basis with your tutor.

If you should have personal problems that prevent you completing the number of observations required, you should discuss this as soon as you can with your tutor. Never be tempted to invent observations or forge signatures. This would undoubtedly lead to you failing the course.

In the placement

Sometimes, in discussion with your supervisor, you will find that you have observed some behaviour or identified a need of which the placement has not been aware. Your observations might then become part of planning an individual programme for the child to help overcome the problem. Occasionally, students' observations have been used at case conferences and have helped to identify issues concerning child protection. In other cases, observations have pointed out that a young child is reading fluently and encouragement can then be given to the child to extend this skill.

Since the Education Reform Act of 1988, which set out the National Curriculum, all educational establishments are required to keep records and assessments of children at a number of key stages, and you may be asked for a copy of some observations to be placed in the child's file. The Education Act of 1981 initiated statements of special educational need, and your observations may be used for helping with assessment.

Sometimes a placement might not always display good practice in one particular area and this might be demonstrated in your observation. You will then have to make a difficult decision as to whether to show this observation to your supervisor or not. If you have any suspicion that any child might be at risk, the best policy would be to discuss the observation with your supervisor/tutor and ask for guidance and advice.

Objectivity

You have learned not to be subjective when writing and interpreting
your observations. Always avoid stereotyping children when setting up
structured observations and when taking part in general discussion in
the placement. For example, if asked by your college to observe doll
play, you would make sure that you did not only invite the girls to take
part. Beware of preconceptions; for example of a child who comes from
a family with multiple problems and is observed exhibiting aggressive
behaviour. A parent may remark, 'What can you expect? His brothers
were just the same'. Do not fall into the trap of scapegoating this child
or indulging in gossip.

Sharing information

All of your observations will be seen by your supervisor and tutor, and
you might want to share some observations with parent/carers. You will
need to work with parent/carers when carrying out longitudinal studies,
as there are obviously periods of time when the child is not in the
placement and you might want to know, for example, how the child
spends the rest of the time at home, what his or her appetite is like, and
how well he or she sleeps. If the child is going through a period when his
or her behaviour is erratic, it is essential to discuss this with the
parent/carer and with your supervisor, so that you can all act together to
help the child.

You must always be aware of the issue of confidentiality, and some
observations should not be generally available to all staff in the
placement. If in doubt, your supervisor will provide guidance.

Occasionally, observations will be seen by other professional workers
outside the placement. For example, language samples might be very
useful to speech therapists. You should only do this with the knowledge
and permission of the supervisor. Professional people all act within their
code of professional conduct and obviously understand the need for
confidentiality.

Compiling a file

For many students, your observation folder will be assessed by the external moderator towards the end of your training. The material must be easy for the moderator to read and follow and therefore you need to organise your work systematically. Regular completion of the observation checklist will allow you to monitor your progress. Routinely, look at your file and count the total of completed observations across the age and technique range. 'Completed' observations are those signed by your supervisor and tutor. At the same time, count the number signed by your supervisor, but not yet handed back to you by your tutor, and the number of observations that you have in rough form still to be written up. The observation checklist allows you to see at a glance where you might have to do further observations.

Moderators are looking for evidence that you have a true understanding of children's normal development, and that your interpretations demonstrate a sensitivity to children's needs. Any observations that show stereotypical attitudes or inappropriate assessments, most likely to be found at the beginning of the course, should be removed from the file.

Although there is no specified number of observations and assessments that have to be completed, there are other constraints, such as the need to cover a range of methods and types of observation. It is unlikely that less than forty-five observations will meet these conditions and, depending on how the task is approached, significantly more than this number of observations may be required. Aiming for a higher number will allow you to destroy some observations that you feel are not up to standard.

Observation Checklist

Date:

Age group	Total signed by supervisor/tutor	Total signed by supervisor and handed in	No. to be written up	Total
0 to 1 year				
1 to 4 years				
4 to 7 years				
Other				
Types of observations				
Written record				
Time sample				
Event sample				
Pie chart				
Bar graph				
Language tape				
Baby study				
Pre-school assessment				
Development guide				
Other longitudinal study				
Target child				
Group observation				
Individual observation				
Sociograms				
Outside placement observation				
Other				

You may photocopy this sheet for your own use. © Stanley Thornes (Publishers) Ltd 1994

Presentation

Observations should be presented in a plain ring folder with your registration and centre numbers only on the outside of the file. Similar paper should be used throughout and it is tidier to use the same colour ink. Many students like to put observations into plastic pockets. Although this keeps them clean and tidy whilst you are storing them, it is not necessary to present them like this in your completed file. In addition to being expensive, it makes the file bulky and sometimes unwieldy to handle. If you have access to a word processor you may prefer to present all or some of your observations typed. Handwritten observations are quite acceptable as long as there are not too many corrected errors and the handwriting is legible. You might find it better to re-write some of your observations rather than offer untidy, messy work. However good the content, giving the moderator a difficult task in reading them will not be in your favour.

It is a good idea to incorporate dividers into the file. They could be used to divide your observations into types of placement, for example 'Nursery school', 'Private family', etc., or into ages, 0 to 1, 1 to 4, 4 to 7 years. This will help people to use the file and find the age group or placement more easily. All observations should have a standard front page.

All observations must be numbered and in date order within the divisions. This will demonstrate the progress you have made. A table of contents is essential.

A matrix must be included and some observations will be recorded more than once as they cover several aspects of development and behaviour. Keeping your matrix up-to-date will help ensure that you cover the full range of observations across the whole age range.

DIPLOMA IN NURSERY NURSING
TABLE OF CONTENTS OF OBSERVATION PORTFOLIO

Observation number	Date	Aim	Age(s) gender	Details of setting	Techniques	Individual/ group
1	11.10.94	Emot. dev.	4:2 M	Bathroom	Written record	I
2	13.10.94	Physical skills	3:6 F	Outside area	"	I
3	25.10.94	Lang. dev.	4:1 F 4:2 F 4:6 F	Class-room	"	G
4	25.10.94	Fine phys dev.	3:6 M	Class room	"	I
5	7.11.94 + 8.11.94	Emot. dev.	4:6 F	Nursery class	Time Sample	I
6	22.11.94	Physical skills	3:2 M	"	Checklist	I

DIPLOMA IN NURSERY NURSING
TABLE OF CONTENTS OF OBSERVATION PORTFOLIO

Observation number	Date	Aim	Age(s) gender	Details of setting	Techniques	Individual/ group

You may photocopy this sheet for your own use. © Stanley Thornes (Publishers) Ltd 1994

Example of a college matrix

Age range (0–4 yr)							Age range (1–4 yrs)					Age range (4–7 yrs)						
0 to 6 weeks	6 weeks to 3 months	3 to 6 months	6 to 9 months	9 months to 1 year	1 year to 18 months	18 months to 2 years	2 to 2.5 years	2.5 to 3 years	3 to 3.5 years	3.5 to 4 years	4 to 4.5 years	4.5 to 5 years	5 to 5.5 years	5.5 to 6 years	6 to 6.5 years	6.5 to 7 years	7 to 8 years	Category
																		Gross motor development
																		Fine/hand-eye co-ordination/manipulation
																		Non-verbal communication
																		Language development
																		Emotional development
																		Patterns of behaviour
																		Relationships with children
																		Relationships with adults
																		Cognitive development
																		Early numeracy
																		Early science
																		Early literacy
																		Problem solving
																		National curriculum
																		Outdoor activities
																		Outings
																		Messy play
																		Creative skills
																		Imaginative skills
																		Small construction
																		Large construction
																		Art
																		Music
																		Health surveillance
																		Care routines
																		Meals/nutrition
																		Accidents
																		Self care
																		Needs
																		Settling in
																		Independence
																		Response of group to individual children
																		Children in a large group
																		Children in a small group

Please indicate observation number in box (it may appear more than once).

Please indicate if it is a group (G) or individual (I) observation, e.g. 1G, 2I, 3I, 4G.

You may photocopy this sheet for your own use. © Stanley Thornes (Publishers) Ltd 1994

THE NATIONAL NURSERY EXAMINATION BOARD

Module A - Observation & Assessment Matrix (Diploma)

Candidate Name: ----------------------   Candidate Number: ----------------

Observation requirements	0 - 1 Year	1 - 4 Years	4 - 7 Years
a) Areas of development:			
physical			
cognitive			
language			
social			
emotional			
b) Learning situations:			
physical skills			
problem solving			
creative skills			
imaginative skills			
others			
c) Types and patterns of behaviour			
d) Physical care and health routines/activities			
e) Indoor situations			
f) Outdoor situations			
g) Group size			
large			
small			
individual child			
h) Care routines			
i) Education routines			
j) Early literacy			
k) Early numeracy			
l) Learning within the National Curriculum			
m) Children with particular needs			
n) Adult/child interation			
o) Child/child interaction			

© NNEB

References/Bibliography

This refers to the reading you have done in order to interpret your observations. At the end of most of your observations you will have put a reference, naming the books and authors which helped you with your analysis. You need to list the books/articles in author alphabetical order, followed by the title of the book or article. For example:

Bee H., *The Developing Child*, Harper & Row, 1978.
Bond S., 'Recording Achievements', Nursery World, 9.9.93.
Roberts M. and Tamburrini J., *Child Development 0–5*, Holmes McDougall, 1981.

When you have completed your file, you may be asked to sign a statement declaring the authenticity of the work.

Using your observations in your future professional role

As a student, you might have initially thought that doing observations was an obstacle that you were expected to surmount in order to gain your qualification. We are confident that by the time you have completed the course you will have become proficient in this skill and be fully informed of how important observing children closely is to your awareness and understanding of their needs and development.

You will find that you will use observations and assessments in many different situations. These will vary from routine to structured assessments in cases of particular need. Observations will help in planning the curriculum and ensuring the most effective use of the learning environment.

Whatever area of child-care employment or future training you enter, observing children will be an integral part of your professional role. Using observations, you will get to know the children in your care in an objective manner and be able to plan suitable routines and individual activities, so as to extend their development and understand total needs. Nursery Nurses are regarded by many other professionals as the experts in using observational techniques and contributing to their interpretation so as to help all children to fulfil their potential.

GOOD PRACTICE FOR THE CHILD-CARE PRACTITIONER

1 Respect confidentiality.
2 Keep files in a secure place.
3 Be ready to share observations and assessments with parent/carers.
4 Be systematic in your recording, making sure that all children are observed regularly.
5 Always be objective.
6 Never jump to conclusions, labelling children, generalising behaviour from one sample or guessing why children respond in a particular manner.
7 Allow for environmental and cultural differences, whilst all the time guarding against racial and sexist attitudes.
8 When directly assessing a child, be careful not to involve yourself in the activity, or to influence the child's behaviour by your manner or tone of voice.
9 Write up your observation notes promptly, so as to give as clear a record as possible of what took place.
10 Use your observations for the benefit of the children and to develop good practice within the workplace.
11 Keep up to date with current research, reading and techniques and be prepared to consider new methods of assessment as they become available.

APPENDIX: DEVELOPMENTAL NORMS

DEVELOPMENTAL NORMS 0 to 1 year

	Physical development – gross motor	Physical development – fine motor	Social and emotional development	Cognitive and language development
At birth	Reflexes: ■ Rooting, sucking and swallowing reflex ■ Grasp reflex ■ Walking reflex ■ Moro reflex If pulled to sit, head falls backwards If held in sitting position, head falls forward, and back is curved In supine (laying on back), limbs are bent In prone (laying on front), lies in fetal position with knees tucked up Unable to raise head or stretch limbs	Reflexes: ■ Pupils reacting to light ■ Opens eyes when held upright ■ Blinks or opens eyes wide to sudden sound ■ Startle reaction to sudden sound ■ Closing eyes to sudden bright light	Bonding/attachment	Cries vigorously, with some variation in pitch and duration
1 month	In prone, lifts chin In supine, head moves to one side. Arm and leg extended on face side Begins to flex upper and lower limbs	Hands fisted Eyes move to dangling objects	Watches mother's face with increasingly alert facial expression Fleeting smile – may be wind! Stops crying when picked up	Cries become more differentiated to indicate needs Stops and attends to voice, rattle and bell
3 months	Held sitting, head straight back and neck firm. Lower back still weak When lying, pelvis is flat	Grasps an object when placed in hand Turns head right round to look at objects Eye contact firmly established	Reacts with pleasure to familiar situations/routines	Regards hands with interest Beginning to vocalise
6 months	In supine, can lift head and shoulders In prone, can raise up on hands Sits with support Kicks strongly May roll over When held, enjoys standing and jumping	Has learned to grasp objects and passes toys from hand to hand Visual sense well established	Takes everything to mouth Responds to different emotional tones of chief caregiver	Finds feet interesting Vocalises tunefully Laughs in play Screams with annoyance Understands purpose of rattle
9 months	Sits unsupported Begins to crawl Pulls to stand, falls back with bump	Visually attentive Grasps with thumb and index finger Releases toy by dropping Looks for fallen objects Beginning to finger-feed Holds bottle or cup	Plays peek-a-boo - can start earlier Imitates hand clapping Clings to familiar adults, reluctant to go to strangers - from about 7 months	Watches activities of others with interest Vocalises to attract attention Beginning to babble Finds partially hidden toy Shows an interest in picture books Knows own name
1 year	Walks holding one hand, may walk alone Bends down and picks up objects Pulls to stand and sits deliberately	Picks up small objects Fine pincer grip Points at objects Holds spoon	Co-operates in dressing Demonstrates affection Participates in nursery rhymes Waves bye bye	Uses jargon Responds to simple instructions and understands several words Puts wooden cubes in and out of cup or box

1 to 4 years

	Physical development – gross motor	Physical development – fine motor	Social and emotional development	Cognitive and language development
1 year	Walks holding one hand, may walk alone Bends down and picks up objects Pulls to stand and sits deliberately	Picks up small objects Fine pincer grip Points at objects Holds spoon	Co-operates in dressing Demonstrates affection Participates in nursery rhymes Waves bye bye	Uses jargon Responds to simple instructions and understands several words Puts wooden cubes in and out of cup or box
15 months	Walking usually well established Can crawl up stairs frontwards and down stairs backwards Kneels unaided Balance poor, falls heavily	Holds crayon with palmar grasp Precise pincer grasp, both hands Builds tower of 2 cubes Can place objects precisely Uses spoon which sometimes rotates Turns pages of picture book	Indicates wet or soiled pants Helps with dressing Emotionally dependent on familiar adult	Jabbers loudly and freely, with 2–6 recognisable words, and can communicate needs Intensely curious Reproduces lines drawn by adult
18 months	Climbs up and down stairs with hand held Runs carefully Pushes, pulls and carries large toys Backs into small chair Can squat to pick up toys	Builds tower of 3 cubes Scribbles to and fro spontaneously Begins to show preference for one hand Drinks without spilling	Tries to sing Imitates domestic activities Bowel control sometimes attained Alternates between clinging and resistance Plays contentedly alone near familiar adult	Enjoys simple picture books, recognising some characters Jabbering established 6–20 recognisable words May use echolalia (repeating adult's last word, or last word of rhyme) Is able to show several parts of the body, when asked Explores environment energetically
2 years	Runs with confidence, avoiding obstacles Walks up and down stairs both feet to each step, holding wall Squats with ease. Rises without using hands Can climb up on furniture and get down again Steers tricycle pushing along with feet Throws small ball overarm, and kicks large ball	Turns picture book pages one at a time Builds tower of 6 cubes Holds pencil with first 2 fingers and thumb near to point	Competently spoon feeds and drinks from cup Is aware of physical needs Can put on shoes and hat Keenly interested in outside environment – unaware of dangers Demands chief caregiver's attention and often clings Parallel play Throws tantrums if frustrated	Identifies photographs of familiar adults Identifies small world toys Recognises tiny details in pictures Uses own name to refer to self Speaks in 2- and 3-word sentences, and can sustain short conversations Asks for names and labels Talks to self continuously

continued

to 4 years *continued*

	Physical development – gross motor	Physical development – fine motor	Social and emotional development	Cognitive and language development
3 years	Competent locomotive skills Can jump off lower steps Still uses 2 feet to a step coming down stairs Pedals and steers tricycle	Cuts paper with scissors Builds a tower of 9 cubes and a bridge with 3 cubes Good pencil control Can thread 3 large beads on a string	Uses spoon and fork Increased independence in self care Dry day and night Affectionate and co-operative Plays co-operatively, particularly domestic play Tries to please	Can copy a circle and some letters Can draw a person with a head and 2 other parts of the body May name colours and match 3 primary colours Speech and comprehension well established Some immature pronunciations and unconventional grammatical forms Asks questions constantly Can give full name, gender and age Relates present activities and past experiences Increasing interest in words and numbers
4 years	All motor muscles well controlled Can turn sharp corners when running Hops on favoured foot Balances for 3–5 seconds Increasing skill at ball games Sits with knees crossed	Builds a tower of 10 cubes Uses 6 cubes to build 3 steps, when shown	Boasts and is bossy Sense of humour developing Cheeky, answers back Wants to be independent Plans games co-operatively Argues with other children but learning to share	Draws person with head, legs and trunk Draws recognisable house Uses correct grammar most of the time Most pronunciations mature Asks meanings of words Enjoys verses and jokes, and may use swear words Counts up to 20 Imaginative play well developed

4 to 7 years

	Physical development – gross motor	Physical development – fine motor	Social and emotional development	Cognitive and language development
4 years	All motor muscles well controlled Can turn sharp corners when running Hops on favoured foot Balances for 3–5 seconds Increasing skill at ball games Sits with knees crossed	Builds a tower of 10 cubes Uses 6 cubes to build 3 steps, when shown	Boasts and is bossy Sense of humour developing Cheeky, answers back Wants to be independent Plans games co-operatively Argues with other children but learning to share	Draws person with head, legs and trunk Draws recognisable house Uses correct grammar most of the time Most pronunciations mature Asks meanings of words Enjoys verses and jokes, and may use swear words Counts up to 20 Imaginative play well developed
5 years	Can touch toes keeping legs straight Hops on either foot Skips Runs on toes Ball skills developing well Can walk along a thin line	Threads needle and sews Builds steps with 3–4 cubes Colours pictures carefully Can copy adult writing	Copes well with daily personal needs Chooses own friends Well-balanced and sociable Sense of fair play and understanding of rules developing Shows caring attitudes towards others	Matches most colours Copies square, triangle and several letters, writing some unprompted Writes name Draws a detailed person Speaks correctly and fluently Knows home address Able and willing to complete projects Understands numbers using concrete objects Imaginary play now involves make-believe games
6 years	Jumps over rope 25 cm high Learning to skip with rope	Ties own shoe laces	Eager for fresh experiences More demanding and stubborn, less sociable Joining a 'gang' may be important May be quarrelsome with friends Needs to succeed as failing too often leads to poor self-esteem	Reading skills developing well Drawings more precise and detailed Figure may be drawn in profile Can describe how one object differs from another Mathematical skills developing, may use symbols instead of concrete objects May write independently
7 years	Rides a 2-wheel bicycle Improved balance	Skills constantly improving More dexterity and precision in all areas	Special friend at school Peer approval becoming important Likes to spend some time alone Enjoys TV and books May be moody May attempt tasks too complex to complete	Moving towards abstract thought Able to read Can give opposite meanings Able to write a paragraph independently